Pediatric Certification Review

Janice Selekman
Louise Jakubik

Janice Selekman, DNSc, RN
Professor
University of Delaware
Newark, Delaware

Louise D. Jakubik, MSN, CRNP, APRN, BC
President and Chief Learning Officer
Nurse Builders
Philadelphia, Pennsylvania

Reviewers:

Lynn Mohr, MS, APRN, BC, CPN
Pediatric Clinical Nurse Specialist
Advocate Hope Children's Hospital
Oak Lawn, Illinois

Aris Beoglos, PhD, RN
Director, Center for Excellence in Nursing Education
Akron Children's Hospital
Akron, Ohio

Dedication:
To pediatric nurses who strive to be the best they can be!

Table of Contents

Society of Pediatric Nurses

NOTICE

CHAPTER

1

Introduction to
Pediatric Nursing Certification Review

LEARNING OBJECTIVES

1. Describe the purpose of pediatric nursing certification.

2. List the benefits of pediatric nursing certification.

3. Identify the two different pediatric nursing certification examinations currently available.

4. Discuss the scoring methods for pediatric nursing certification examinations.

5. Identify preparation resources and strategies for pediatric nursing certification examinations.

I. Introduction to *Pediatric Nursing Certification Review*

This book is designed to be a key resource as you prepare to take a pediatric nursing certification examination. The text provides an overview of pediatric nursing content for the pediatric nurse with a minimum of 1 year of full-time experience in pediatric nursing, or the equivalent within the past 3 to 4 years, depending on the examination requirements.

II. Pediatric nursing certification: Overview

- A. Description
    1. Achievement of pediatric nursing certification is a professional milestone that signifies the attainment of a core body of knowledge in pediatric nursing beyond the basic or entry level.
    2. The two certification examinations described in this book are nationally recognized examinations developed by content experts in the field of pediatric nursing.
- B. Certification organizations
    1. Certification organizations develop and implement certification exams and set prerequisite requirements such as hours of practice experience and educational preparation.
    2. There are two certification boards that offer national certification in pediatric nursing: the Pediatric Nursing Certification Board (PNCB) and the American Nurses Credentialing Center (ANCC).
    3. Each certification organization publishes an exam content outline that delineates the number of questions that appear on the exam in specific content areas.
    4. Information about the specific examinations is available by contacting the certification organizations directly or by visiting their Web sites.
        - *a)* Pediatric Nursing Certification Board—www.pncb.org
        - *b)* American Nurses Credentialing Center—www. nursingworld.org
- C. Exam requirements and content
    1. Exams require a minimum of 1-2 years experience over the past 3 to 4 years as an RN in a pediatric nursing specialty, or equivalent experience.
    2. Both cover the application of the nursing process that covers the spectrum from health promotion and disease prevention to illness management for acute and chronic conditions.

3. Both cover the physical and psychosocial needs of children from infancy through adolescence.
4. Both cover the care of children in a variety of settings, including inpatient acute and long-term care settings, outpatient clinics, community sites, the schools, and the home.
5. Both have a heavy focus on growth and development of the child and family-centered care.

D. Purpose and benefits
1. Specialty certification in pediatric nursing is a career milestone for the individual nurse and a sign of distinction for organizations that employ a certified nursing workforce.
    a) Individual benefits
        (1) Nurses who achieve certification demonstrate attainment of a core body of knowledge to enhance their practice as pediatric nurses.
        (2) The individual benefits of pediatric nursing certification include but are not limited to
            (a) Increased confidence in clinical decision making
            (b) Professional recognition
            (c) Career advancement
2. Organizational benefits
    a) Organizations that have facilitated the achievement of a largely certified pediatric nursing workforce have reported benefits such as
        (1) Institutional recognition
    b) Improved ability to meet organizational goals such as external recognition and accreditation

E. Scoring methods
1. Certification exam scoring is on a pass/fail basis.
2. The exam is a criterion-referenced exam, meaning that achievement of a set minimum score, called the cut score, signifies that the exam taker has demonstrated a core body of knowledge necessary to pass the exam.

F. Preparation resources and strategies
1. Preparation for taking a pediatric nursing certification exam is an individualized process. There are, however, some general rules that may assist you in your studying.
    a) Identify your areas of content strength and weakness based on the content outline of the pediatric nursing certification exam you are choosing to take.

        (1) Your areas of strength are those areas that require little or no study time.

        (2) Your areas of weakness are the content areas on which you will focus your study time.

  b) Identify an approach to studying that will work for you.

        (1) Individual study

        (2) Partnered study (study with another pediatric nurse preparing for the exam)

        (3) Group study (study with a group of nurses preparing for the exam, such as a group from your unit or hospital)

  c) Identify a timeline/schedule for studying that will keep you focused and motivated.

        (1) Daily

            (*a*) A small amount of studying each day can be motivating and make the study process seem less overwhelming.

        (2) Weekly

            (*a*) Choosing a block of time to study once or twice per week can be a useful way to schedule quality study time with no interruptions.

  d) Take practice tests as often as possible.

        (1) Practice test questions are a key strategy to get you familiar with the test-taking process, as well as to reinforce content information.

        (2) Use the specific chapter practice questions at the end of this book after studying each chapter to test your content knowledge.

CHAPTER
2

Overview of Pediatric Nursing

LEARNING OBJECTIVES

1. Describe the scope of pediatric nursing.
2. Discuss the principles of family-centered care and their practice implications.

I. Scope of pediatric nursing

Pediatric nursing is a nursing specialty that involves the care of children from birth through adolescence (0 to 18 years) and their families. Pediatric nurses practice in a variety of settings including communities, schools, clinics, and hospital settings. The continuum of pediatric nursing extends from health and wellness to death and dying. Across the continuum of care, the focus of pediatric nursing includes health promotion and injury/disease prevention, acute and chronic conditions, and end-of-life and palliative care.

II. Family-centered care

A. Overview

Family-centered care, treating the family as a unit, provides the philosophical foundation for pediatric nursing practice. Guiding principles for family-centered care include partnership, information sharing, participation, and collaboration. Lewandowski and Tesler (2003) outlined evidence-based practice recommendations for the eight elements of family-centered care.

Family-centered care element	Description	Practice recommendations
Family as the center	The family is the center and constant in the child's life. The healthcare delivery system and healthcare providers fluctuate. The entire family system is affected by the child's illness or injury.	Comprehensive family assessments Sibling and extended family member involvement
Family-professional collaboration	Families are partners in the health care of their children.	Mutual goal setting Mutual decision making Parental presence and access • 24-hour access • Presence in procedures Parental participation in • Institutional and community program development • Advisory boards • Policy development and evaluation

Family-professional communication	Information exchange with families should be complete, unbiased, and supportive.	Promote mutual (two-way) communication and family input.
Cultural diversity of families	Policies and practices exist that recognize and respect the diversity of families in terms of a variety of differences including ethnicity, race, spirituality, cultural norms and customs, economic and educational background, and the home and community environment.	Provide culturally competent care. Respect and support family beliefs and practices. Provide equitable quality and access to health care.
Coping differences and supports	Recognize that families have a variety of coping mechanisms and support systems.	Provide policies and programs that recognize the diverse coping needs of families. Promote healthcare providers' roles in supporting family coping factors to include <ul><li>Assess strengths and weaknesses of coping mechanisms among families.</li><li>Support resiliency factors.</li><li>Identify maladaptive coping mechanisms.</li><li>Assist families in modifying coping methods.</li><li>Respect and support differences in coping.</li></ul> Provide formal and informal support mechanisms for families.
Family-centered peer support	Encourage and facilitate family-to-family support and networking.	Provide information for families regarding formal and informal family-to-family support. Create and promote psychoeducational groups for parents, siblings, and the ill/injured child.

Specialized service and support systems	Provide and promote care for children with specialized health and developmental care needs that are flexible, accessible, and comprehensive.	Provide comprehensive and coordinated services. Provide case management and care coordination across healthcare settings, the community, and the home. Create and promote advocacy roles for healthcare providers.
Holistic perspective of family-centered care	Recognize the child and family as a whole. Understand that health care is only one facet of the child's and family's life.	Promote normal developmental milestones. Encourage identities beyond the illness state. Promote normalization among family members and the family as a unit.

Note. From Lewandowski & Tesler (2003).

   B.   Nursing care issues
      1.   Sibling involvement
         a)   Involve siblings in care based on their developmental level.
         b)   Remember that the older preschool age and younger school-age siblings may have magical thinking, believing that it is their fault that their sibling is ill or hospitalized.
            (1)   Use active listening techniques.
            (2)   Provide siblings with support groups.
         c)   Consider that the child's acute or chronic condition affects the entire family system, influencing the parents' ability to provide care and attention to well siblings.
            (1)   Well siblings may have abrupt changes to their normal routines as a result of a sibling's illness or hospitalization.
      2.   Family presence/visitation
         a)   Parents should have 24-hour access to the hospitalized child.
            (1)   Involve parents in patient rounds.
            (2)   Provide sleeping accommodations for the parent at patient's bedside.
      3.   End-of-life/emergency care

        a) Promote parental presence during procedures and cardiopulmonary (CPR) resuscitation; evidence demonstrates that presence assists the patient's coping, promotes communication and partnership with families, and facilitates the bereavement process among families of children who have died as a result of the inability to resuscitate.

    4. Shift-to-shift report/rounds

        a) Be aware of the negative effects of "labeling" patients and families in the family-centered care process, because labels work against partnership and collaboration with patients and families.

        b) Promote opportunities to include parents in interdisciplinary rounds; this encourages partnership and mutual information sharing.

III. The spectrum of care

  A. Pediatric nursing involves the entire health continuum, from wellness through acute illness and chronic conditions.

  B. Health promotion is key to attaining and maintaining a state of good overall health.

    1. For children, the focus is on the following:

        a) Nutrition

        b) Personal hygiene

        c) Exercise

        d) Sleep and rest

        e) Dental care

        f) Being cared for and about

        g) Stimulating the mind

        h) Keeping safe

    2. These are promoted by

        a) Well-child care visits to the health care provider

        b) Anticipatory guidance to parents

        c) Education to children and adolescents

        d) Height, weight, hearing, vision, blood pressure, and posture screening

  C. Disease prevention

    1. Screen to detect disease or alterations in health and development early in their occurrence; examples are

        a) Developmental screenings for high-risk children

        b) Screening for tuberculosis

    2. Immunizations

D. Acute disease management
1. The earlier the disease is detected and treated, in general, the less morbidity that results.
2. There is a spectrum of acute disease from mild (outpatient) to moderate (inpatient) to serious (critical care).
3. Acute disease usually resolves but can be fatal or lead to serious complications.

E. Chronic conditions
1. A chronic condition is one that lasts at least 6 months; it may be relatively permanent and may result in limitations in the activities of daily living
2. Chronic conditions may be due to the following:
   a) Genetic or congenital conditions
   b) Autoimmune disease
   c) Organ failure
   d) Trauma
   e) Cancer
   f) Psychological conditions
3. Chronic conditions may result from the consequences of the following
   a) Prematurity
   b) Infection
   c) High-risk behaviors
4. Any chronic condition can affect the child's physical, psychological, and social growth and development.
5. Chronic conditions have a psychological impact on all members of the family.
6. Focus on the child's strengths; stress what is special in each child; provide as much autonomy as possible.
7. Normalize the child's environment; provide normal childhood experiences, even for a child connected to high-technology equipment; provide consistent limits, rules, and routines; promote growth and development.
8. Provide rehabilitation/habilitation, if warranted.
9. Federal laws provide rights to a free education, access, and accommodations (see Chapter 18).

Reference

Lewandowski, L.A., & Tesler, M.D. (2003). *Family centered care: Putting it into action: The SPN/ANA guide to family-centered care.* Washington, DC: nursesbooks.org

CHAPTER

3

Growth and Development

LEARNING OBJECTIVES

1. Discuss the major concepts associated with growth and development, and describe their impact on pediatric nursing.

2. Identify the physical, psychosocial, and cognitive developmental tasks for the child from birth through adolescence.

3. Plan developmentally-based nursing care strategies that promote anticipatory guidance and injury prevention.

4. Determine the child's nutrition and safety needs.

5. Identify behavioral reactions to illness and hospitalization in the child from birth through adolescence.

6. Identify common issues in the parent-child relationship from birth through adolescence.

7. Plan communication techniques and other nursing interventions based on the child's needs and ability to comprehend.

I. Chapter overview

A. The concepts of growth and development are fundamental to the practice of pediatric nursing. Throughout the periods of child development, major milestones are accomplished. Developmentally appropriate approaches to nursing care require an understanding of each of these developmental periods.

B. All interventions are based on the following principles:
1. All interventions are family-centered, treating the child and family as a unit.
2. The goal is to help the child and family unit attain, maintain, or regain optimal health.
3. Nursing interventions are guided by both the child's chronologic age and level of development (physical and mental).
4. Health and development are affected by environment and heredity.

II. Introduction: Concepts of growth and development

A. Growth and development are not synonymous.
1. Growth implies an increase in size but does not necessarily include development.
2. Development describes the maturation of structures and includes growth.
3. Parents need to be taught the normal childhood growth and development parameters.

B. Growth and development progress in three ways.
1. From head to toe (cephalocaudally)
2. From the trunk to the tips of the extremities (proximodistally)
3. From the general to the specific (for example, progressing from crawling to walking to skipping)

C. Growth follows an orderly and predictable pattern during developmental periods.
1. Infancy (birth to 12-15 months)—a period of rapid growth in which the head grows faster than other tissues
2. Toddler-preschool age (12-15 months to 5 years)—a period of slow growth in which the trunk grows faster
3. School age (5-12 years)—a period of slow growth in which the limbs grow fastest
4. Adolescence (13-20 years)—a period of rapid growth for the trunk, including the gonads and associated tissues

D. A developmental assessment determines whether the child has mastered certain expected accomplishments during a developmental stage; if not, subsequent tasks may be delayed.
   1. Development is assessed on a continuum throughout childhood.
   2. Typically, development is assessed by using a combination of parent history taking and gross assessment by the nurse and/or the primary care provider.

III. Theories of development

Theories of child development provide a basis for how we understand the development of personality (Erikson), cognition (Piaget), and morality (Kohlberg). Each theory measures a *different* component of development.

A. Psychosocial development: Erikson
   Erik Erikson's psychosocial-based theory is the most commonly accepted model for child development, although it cannot be empirically tested. Each stage has a core conflict to be resolved by individuals and an outcome goal for healthy personality development.

Erikson (Psychosocial Development)

Age	Stage	Stage description
Infancy (0 to 12-18 months)	**Trust versus mistrust**	Trust is essential for development of a healthy personality and is fostered by consistent and loving care from a consistent, caring figure. Consistency allows the infant to predict responses.
		Mistrust is promoted when trust-promoting experiences are not present and when basic needs are inconsistently or inadequately met.
		Virtue/psychological strength being developed: **Hope**
Toddlerhood (1-3 years)	**Autonomy versus shame and doubt**	Autonomy is fostered through the freedom and encouragement to master new things and become independent related to himself/herself and the environment. Shame and doubt are promoted when overdependency is fostered where independence is possible; the child is made to feel self-conscious, or his/her independent decisions have negative consequences.
		Virtue/psychological strength being developed: **Will**

Early childhood (3-6 years)	**Initiative versus guilt**	The conscience develops here when a child recognizes the guidance of not only outsiders but also an "inner voice." The focus is maintaining a sense of initiative without impinging on the rights and privileges of others or developing an overwhelming sense of guilt. Virtue/psychological strength being developed: **Purpose**
Middle childhood (6-12 years)	**Industry versus inferiority**	The focus here is on achievement. Competition and cooperation with others is an important component of this stage; learning rules is also important. This stage is marked by social relationships. Inferiority or inadequacy occurs when a child is unable to meet others' expectations or if he/she feels that external standards are too high. Virtue/psychological strength being developed: **Competence**
Adolescence (12-19 years)	**Identity versus role confusion**	The child's body is rapidly changing. He/she becomes concerned with others' opinions as compared with his/her own sense of self-concept. Identification of roles and integration of own values with society are key issues. An important milestone includes decision making regarding a future occupation. Inability to resolve these conflicts results in role confusion. Virtue/psychological strength being developed: **Fidelity/loyalty**

B. Cognitive development: Piaget

Jean Piaget's theory of cognitive development is concerned with the child's cognitive development through interaction with the environment. Each stage involves a mental activity; these occur in an orderly and sequential fashion.

Piaget (Cognitive Development)

Stage/age	Stage	Stage description
Birth to 2 years	**Sensorimotor**	Intellectual development occurs through the child's interaction with the environment. Progression is from reflexive behavior to simple, repetitive behavior to imitative behavior. A sense of time and space develops with routines, and a sense of cause and effect develops. Object permanence is eventually recognized here, and language development begins to occur.
2 to 7 years	**Preoperational** (preconceptual = 2-4 years; intuitive = 4-7 years)	Egocentrism is the primary element of cognitive development. The child is unable to see things from any perspective other than his/her own. Thinking is magical, concrete, and dominated by perception; it is done in a nonlogical and nonreversible manner. Reasoning becomes intuitive and transducive (infers particulars from particulars, rather than inductive or deductive). Uses symbols, language, and imitation to learn.
7-11 years	**Concrete operations**	Thought becomes more logical. Thinking is in terms of the world as concrete and tangible. The child develops a sense of conservation and reversibility. Reasoning is inductive; masters facts and collects and sorts objects. The child is able to consider others' points of view.
11-15 years	**Formal operations**	Adaptability and flexibility developed here. Abstract thought develops. New ideas can be created and situations can be analyzed.

    C. Moral development: Kohlberg
        Kohlberg's theory describes the development of morality according to the principles of cognitive developmental theory.

Kohlberg (Moral Development)

Age	Level	Description
Toddlerhood and early childhood	**Preconventional or premoral**	This stage is characterized by a child's conformity to rules that are imposed by authority figures. Stage begins with behavior that is guided by the avoidance of punishment. Later, behavior is guided by reward or other positive reinforcement of desired behavior.
Middle childhood	**Conventional**	This stage is characterized by social conformity and loyalty. Initially, the child seeks approval. Later, the child seeks to avoid "getting in trouble" or getting caught.
Adolescence	**Post-conventional**	This stage is characterized by the child's adoption of his/her own set of moral principles and values. These principles serve to guide a child's individual standards of behavior.

IV. Cultural implications

A. Culture is often the context in which children and their families interpret wellness and the cause, presence, and prognosis of illness.

B. Culture may determine one's use of recommended prevention measures and the interventions one may find acceptable, such as diet.

C. Communication styles (e.g., whether or not eye contact or touch is acceptable), food customs (e.g., keeping kosher or being a vegetarian), and who the decision maker is are all influenced by culture.

D. It is essential for the pediatric nurse to assess the cultural components that are important to a family before making judgments or developing a plan of care.

V. Assessment and measurement of growth and development

A. Growth principles

1. Weight
   a) Normal patterns and rate
      (1) Average newborn: 7 lb
         (a) Maternal nutrition and genetics influence birth weight.
      (2) 5 Months: double birth weight
      (3) 1 Year: triple birth weight
      (4) After 1 year
         (a) Weight after 1 year is largely a result of environmental influences, such as diet and physical activity level; it is also influenced by one's health.
   b) Body mass index (BMI)
      (1) BMI is the recommended method for screening children for overweight and underweight; it correlates weight and height for age on a chart using percentiles.
      (2) BMI in children is gender and age specific.
      (3) BMI can be used beginning at 2 years and tracked through adulthood.
      (4) BMI parameters in children and adolescents indicate the following:
         (a) ≥95% = Overweight
         (b) 85%-<95% = At risk for overweight
         (c) <5% = Underweight
   c) Measurement techniques
      (1) Weigh infants and children <2 years naked on an infant scale.
         (a) Greater accuracy is obtained by using an infant scale.
         (b) Lay infant down to weigh; place in sitting position when this skill is mastered, keeping his or her legs on the scale.
         (c) Keep a hand an inch away from the child to prevent falls.
      (2) Weigh children >2 years of age on a standing scale wearing a gown or light clothing.
         (a) Ensure safety while the child is on the scale.
         (b) Calibrate or zero the scale daily.
         (c) Weigh on the same scale for subsequent visits.
         (d) Document the weight in kilograms, as well as pounds.

2. Length/height
    a) Normal growth rates
        (1) Average newborn: 20 in.
        (2) Growth in first year: 10 in.
        (3) Growth in second year: 5 in.
        (4) Growth each year from age 2 to puberty: 2.5 in.
    b) Birth length doubles at 4 years of age
    c) Linear growth measurement at age 2 years is roughly half of the child's adult height.
    d) Measurement techniques
        (1) Length
            (a) Assessment of a child's length requires the use of a length board. A length board can be used for a child up to age 36 months and plotted on the corresponding 0 to 36 months length growth chart.
        (2) Height
            (a) Assessment of a child's height requires the use of a stadiometer. A standing height can be taken on a child who is able to stand and follow directions beginning at age 24 months. Children younger than 24 months should not be measured standing because the height growth chart does not include children under 2 years.
            (b) When standing, children should be measured while standing against a hard surface; their heels, buttocks, shoulders, and head should make contact with the surface.
            (c) Chart height in centimeters, as well as inches.

 ALERT: Children under 36 months who are measured standing up and whose height is then plotted on a length growth chart will appear proportionally shorter. Conversely, children over 24 months whose length is measured and then plotted on a height growth chart will appear disproportionately taller. The reason for this is that infants and toddlers have an exaggerated lumbar lordosis (curvature), which straightens when they lie down for linear growth assessment.

3. Head circumference
   a) Growth principles
      (1) Head circumference is an important indication of brain growth.
      (2) The brain grows fastest during infancy and early toddlerhood, but continues to grow until 18 years of age.
      (3) Head size is disproportionately large among infants and toddlers.
   b) Measurement
      (1) Measure the head circumference in children up to 36 months of age using a paper tape measure (one that will not stretch).
      (2) Place the tape measure over the brow and around the most prominent portion of the head to obtain the largest head circumference.
   c) Documentation
      (1) Document the head circumference on the appropriate growth chart.

VI. Growth charts

A. Growth charts
   1. Charts were revised in 2000. Changes include the combination of breast-fed and formula-fed infants and the addition of the BMI beginning at 2 years to replace the weight for height assessment.
   2. Measurements are recorded as percentiles of height for age, weight for age, head circumference for age, and BMI.
   3. Findings that require further evaluation include crossing multiple percentiles over a short period of time, measurement at or below the 5th percentile, and a BMI of greater than 85%.

B. Documentation
   1. Selecting the appropriate growth chart
      a) Birth to 36 months (male and female)—a "length" chart
         (1) Children birth to 24 months *must* use this chart.
         (2) Children 24 months to 36 months who are measured *lying down must* use this chart.
   2. 2 Years to 20 years (male and female)—a "height" chart
      a) Children 3 years to 18 years *must* use this chart.
      b) Children 24 months to 36 months who are measured *standing up must* use this chart.

VII. Vital signs

A. Temperature
   1. Oral thermometers are not used until after age 4 to 5 years.
   2. Rectal temperature is approximately 1 °C higher and axillary temperatures are approximately 1°C lower than oral temperature, but these values vary.
   3. A temperature below 38 °C (100.4 °F) is not considered a fever; some use 101 °F as the cutoff for fever management, unless the child appears unwell.
   4. If tympanic temperature measurement is used, position ear so that the infrared sensor focuses on the eardrum; this may require the ear to be pulled up.
   5. Avoid rectal temperatures in neutropenic patients and after rectal surgery.

B. Respirations
   1. Respiratory rate decreases with age.
   2. Infants are diaphragmatic breathers; their breathing may be irregular, so count for a full minute.
   3. Infants are obligate nose breathers.
   4. Newborn rate = 35/min (range = 32-60/min); 2 years = 25/min; 10 years = 19/min.

C. Pulse
   1. Pulse rates decrease with age.
   2. Take for a full minute in children.
   3. Pulses are graded by ease of palpation from 0 (not palpable) to 4 (strong, bounding, and not obliterated with pressure); normal is 3.
   4. Newborn rate = 110-160 beats/min at rest awake; 2 years = 70-110 beats/min; 10 years = 55-90 beats/min.

D. Blood pressure (BP)
   1. BP increases with age.
   2. BP readings vary with cuff width; a cuff that is too large will yield a lower BP, and a cuff that is too narrow will result in an increased BP.
   3. Bladder width should be 40% of arm circumference midway between the olecranon and the acromion.
   4. The cuff bladder should cover 80% to 100% of the circumference of the arm.
   5. Newborn mean BP = 65/41 mmHg; 2 years = 102/58 mmHg; 12 years = 119/76 mmHg.

VIII. Pain assessment

A. Overview
1. Pain is a symptom that occurs whenever the child says it does; all reports of pain should be taken seriously.
2. Pain has physiologic and psychological components.
   a) The child may associate pain with punishment.
3. Expression of pain is influenced by culture and by child-rearing practices.
4. Pain thresholds vary.
5. Pain assessment is considered the fifth vital sign.

B. Assessment
1. Determine the intensity, type, location, duration, and circumstances of the pain; assess whether the child can be distracted from the pain.
2. Assess for crying, facial grimaces, restlessness, irritability, insomnia, anger, diaphoresis, increased pulse and respiratory rates, decreased interactions and withdrawal, diminished appetite, fatigue, and behavioral changes.
3. Use available pediatric pain assessment scales, based on age and cognitive development. Examples include the following:
   a) CRIES Neonatal Postoperative Pain Measurement Scale
      (1) Measures crying, oxygen saturation, heart rate, BP, expression, sleeplessness
   b) FACES Scale
      (1) Uses pictures of six faces that range from happy because it doesn't hurt to hurts the most.
      (2) Child over age 3 can select the face that best depicts his or her pain.
   c) Visual Analog Scale
      (1) A straight line or a numbered line that goes from no pain to the most pain possible and child identifies the pain level
   d) FLACC Pain Assessment Scale
      (1) For preverbal or nonverbal children
      (2) Assesses the face, legs, activity, cry, and consolability
   e) Numeric Scale
      (1) Using 0 as no pain and 10 as the worst pain imaginable, have the child rate the pain intensity.
      (2) Used for children 8 years and older who understand the concept of numbers.

    C. Interventions
1. Reinforce the fact that pain is not a punishment for misbehavior.
2. Apply comfort measures.
3. Offer distraction, such as reading a story or playing a game; promote guided imagery and positive self-talk.
4. Stay with child; let the child assist in painful procedures, such as helping to remove a bandage, to get a sense of control.
5. Administer pain medication without delay to relieve discomfort.
6. Patient-controlled analgesic (PCA) administration can be used by children as young as 5, or by their parents (proxy-controlled analgesia).
7. Morphine is the standard for severe pain; moderate pain can be managed by nonsteroidal anti-inflammatory drugs (ibuprofen) and opioid analgesics.
8. Use lidocaine/prilocaine sprays or ointments (such as EMLA) before injections or intravenous (IV) starts.
9. Oral sucrose is often used for young infants.
10. Allow child to do to a doll or stuffed animal what is done to him or her.

IX. Principles of age

    A. Chronologic age—years or months since birth date

    B. Mental age—level of cognitive function
1. This is based on at least two different types of intelligence tests administered over 6 months, with the child in optimal health.
2. When the child's mental age and chronologic age differ, provide toys, teach safety, and communicate on the basis of mental age.

    C. Bone age
1. The tarsals and carpals are X-rayed to determine the degree of ossification.
2. The measure is used for the child who is shorter or taller than chronologic age suggests.

    D. Adjusted/corrected age—chronologic age minus number of weeks born prematurely.
1. Prematurity is considered a postgestational age less than 37 weeks.

2. In general, growth charting should be adjusted for prematurity for the first 2 years of life.

X. Development assessment

A. Denver Developmental Screening Tests (Denver II)
A classic developmental screening to assess childhood development is called the Denver II (1992). This is a highly specialized, valid, and reliable method of developmental assessment that measures development for children up to 6 years of age in each of four areas: (1) personal-social, (2) fine motor adaptive, (3) language, and (4) gross motor.
   1. The categories and parameters outlined in the Denver II provide a resource and guide for nursing assessments of developmental milestones using observation and history taking during each health encounter.
   2. The Denver does *not* measure intelligence.
B. Wechsler Intelligence Scale for Children–III (WISC)/Wechsler Preschool and Primary Scale of Intelligence–Revised (WPPSI-R)
   1. WPPSI is for ages 4.5 to 6 years; WISC is for those 6 to 16 years.
   2. These scales result in a full-scale Intelligence Quotient (IQ), a Verbal IQ index, and a Performance IQ index.
C. Bayley Scales of Infant and Toddler Development–III
   1. Measure the cognitive, language, motor, social-emotional, and adaptive behavior domains
   2. Often used to determine development in follow-up assessments of premature infants

XI. Nursing interventions for growth and development: Overview

A. During each health encounter with a child, basic assessment of growth and development would include the following nursing interventions.
   1. Developmental history taking
   2. Developmental screening
   3. Growth measurement
   4. Parent teaching regarding developmental milestones (anticipatory guidance) and what caretakers should do to promote physiologic, cognitive, and psychosocial development and safety

XII. Developmental milestones and approaches to care: Infant (0-12 months)

A. Overview
1. 0 to 3 Months
   a) The neonatal period is the first 28 days of life; it has the highest mortality rate of any period in childhood.
   b) Head circumference and chest circumference are approximately equal at birth, although the head circumference is often larger than the chest circumference by 2 to 3 cm.
   c) Head length is one-fourth that of the total body.
   d) The posterior fontanel closes at approximately 2 months.
   e) The newborn has poor ability to regulate temperature control because of poorly developed sweating and shivering mechanisms. Care should be taken to do the following.
      (1) Limit exposure to the cold during baths.
      (2) Cover the head when the neonate is wet or cold.
      (3) Take measures to limit cold exposure during hospital procedures, such as X-ray.
   f) Hearing and touch are well developed at birth; all infants should have a hearing test in the neonatal period, especially those who are receiving ototoxic medications.
   g) Vision is poor. Black and white are the colors best seen by the neonate. The neonate begins to focus on nearby faces. By 3 months, the infant develops binocular vision; the eyes can follow an object 180°.
2. 4 to 6 Months
   a) Birth weight doubles at 5 months.
   b) Infant
      (1) Becomes more social
      (2) Sleeps through the night with one or two naps a day
      (3) Begins teething (lower central incisors appear first); this may result in increased drooling and irritability
      (4) Explores own feet
      (5) Develops full color vision and improved distance vision
      (6) Develops an improvement in the ability to track objects with the eyes (failure to track objects or respond to sound signifies a need for additional assessments of hearing and vision)

3. 7 to 9 Months
   a) This is a stage of tremendous motor development. Environmental safety is of paramount importance during this age group.
4. 10 to 12 Months
   a) Motor development remains the focus. Environmental safety remains of paramount importance during this age group.
   b) Birth weight triples by 12 months.
   c) Length increases by 50% from birth.

B. Psychosocial development
   1. Trust-promoting experiences are essential during infancy including:
      a) Establishment of attachment to a primary caregiver (usually the mother)
      b) Meeting basic needs such as feeding and comforting when crying

 ALERT: Parents should be assured that they cannot spoil an infant. It is important to hold and comfort a crying infant in order to meet basic needs for establishing trust.

   2. 0 to 3 Months
      a) The infant's instinctual smile develops at 2 months and social smile at 3 months.
         (1) The social smile is the infant's first social response. It initiates social relationships, indicates memory traces, and signals the beginning of thought processes.
      b) The infant recognizes the parent's voice.
      c) The neonate is stimulated by being held or rocked, listening to music, or watching a black and white mobile.
   3. 4 to 6 Months
      a) At 4 months the infant laughs in response to the environment.
      b) The infant cries when the parent leaves; this is a normal sign of attachment.
      c) The infant discerns one face from another and exhibits stranger anxiety (is wary of strangers and clings to or clutches parents).
      d) The infant begins comforting habits such as thumb sucking, rubbing an ear, holding a blanket or stuffed toy.

         (1) All of these habits symbolize parents and security.

         (2) Thumb sucking in infancy does not result in malocclusion of permanent teeth.

  4. 7 to 9 Months

     a) The infant imitates the expressions of others.

     b) The infant likes to look in the mirror.

     c) The infant understands the tone of the word "no"; discipline can begin.

     d) The infant enjoys playing simple games like peek-a-boo, playing with toys that make noise, or listening to music.

  5. 10 to 12 Months

     a) The infant may exhibit marked stranger anxiety.

     b) The infant will test the caregiver's reaction by throwing the bottle or cup off the high chair to test the caregiver's response (e.g., picking it up).

     c) The infant claps hands, waves bye-bye, and enjoys rhythm games.

C. Cognitive development

  1. 0 to 3 Months

     a) Notices own hands

     b) Observes people's faces and watches mobiles

  2. 4 to 6 Months

     a) The infant smiles and laughs in response to pleasant environmental stimuli.

  3. 7 to 9 Months

     a) The infant develops object permanence (a principle from Piaget's theory). The infant searches for objects outside the visual field, knowing that even though the object cannot be seen it is still present. Before an infant develops object permanence, if an object is hidden while the infant watches, the infant will not look for it, as the infant thinks the object is gone because it is out of sight.

  4. 10 to 12 Months

     a) Finds hidden object easily

     b) Points to or looks at correct image when named

     c) Uses simple gestures such as shakes head for "no"

     d) Responds to simple verbal requests (e.g., "Bring mama the ball.")

     e) The infant learns through increased exploration of the environment. Sensorimotor experiences should be positive ones.

D. Language/communication
1. 0 to 3 Months
    a) Begins to babble
    b) Turns head toward sound
    c) Cries to indicate need.
        (1) Respond to those needs in a consistent manner to promote trust.
2. 4 to 6 Months
    a) Responds to own name
    b) Continuous babbling occurs.
    c) Babbles in response to sounds as in a conversation by age 6 months
3. 7 to 9 Months
    a) The infant can say all vowels and most consonants but speaks no intelligible words.
    b) The infant understands the word "no" at 9 months. Use of this word should be limited. Instead, the physical environment should be made safe and secure such that verbal limit setting is an exception rather than a routine.
4. 10 to 12 Months
    a) The infant says "mama" and "dada."
    b) The infant can say about five words but understands many more.
    c) The infant repeats sounds and gestures.
E. Motor skills
1. 0 to 3 Months
    a) All motor behavior is under reflex control at birth; extremities are flexed at birth.
        (1) Reflexes reach a peak at 4 to 8 weeks, especially the sucking reflex, which affords nutrition, survival, and psychological pleasure. (Provide a pacifier.)
    b) When prone, the neonate can lift the head slightly off the bed but not off a pillow. (Do not use pillows in the crib.) By 3 months, lying on stomach, neonate will raise head and chest.
    c) At age 3 months, the most primitive reflexes begin to disappear except for the protective and postural reflexes (the blink, cough, swallow, and gag reflexes), which remain for life.
    d) The posterior fontanel closes at 2 months.
    e) When held, the infant begins to hold up own head.
    f) The infant begins to put hand to mouth.
    g) The infant reaches out voluntarily but is uncoordinated.

2. 4 to 6 Months
   a) The infant first rolls over from stomach to back, then from back to front.
   b) The infant reaches for objects and voluntarily grasps them.
   c) The infant transfers objects from one hand to the other.
   d) The infant rakes objects with hands.
   e) When prone, the infant uses the arms to push the chest up while resting the lower body on the knees. The infant rocks back and forth in this position and may begin to crawl on belly backwards now or in the next developmental stage.
   f) The infant sits with support. May begin to sit without support.
3. 7 to 9 Months
   a) The infant sits alone without assistance.
   b) The infant creeps forward on hands and knees with the belly off the floor (crawls).
   c) The infant stands while holding onto an object for support such as a parent's hand or a table.
   d) The infant develops a pincer grasp and places everything in the mouth.
   e) The infant self-feeds crackers, Cheerios, and a bottle. The infant who is emotionally ready can be weaned to a cup.
4. 10 to 12 Months
   a) The infant cruises at 10 months (sidesteps while holding on).
   b) The infant walks with support at 11 months.
   c) The infant takes first steps at 12 months, with variability up to 15 to 16 months.
   d) The infant claps hands, waves bye-bye, and enjoys rhythm games.
   e) The infant explores everything by feeling, pushing, turning, pulling, biting, smelling, and testing for sound; enjoys cloth books and toys to build with and knock over.

F. Developmental approaches to care of infants
   1. Care
      a) Avoid separating the infant from the parent during care.
      b) Use quiet times while the infant is sleeping or being held by a parent to perform assessments that require the infant to be quiet (cardiac and respiratory).

2. Play
   a) Distract the infant with games such as peek-a-boo and playing with rattles.
3. Teaching
   a) The focus of teaching is the parent. Try to provide time for teaching when the infant is calm or sleeping.
4. Observe for maladaptive responses to illness and hospitalization.
   a) Infant exhibits signs of distress such as irritability, poor feeding, and lack of attachment to others. (Crying on separation from mother is normal.)
5. In the hospital, provide for developmentally supportive nursing interventions:
   a) Encourage parental presence and involvement.
   b) Provide consistency regarding routines and caregivers.
   c) Promote positive sensorimotor experiences.

G. Anticipatory guidance and injury prevention
   1. 0 to 3 Months
      a) Crib safety: Soft pillows, crib bumpers, blankets, and stuffed animals should not be placed in the crib as they pose suffocation hazards for the neonate.
      b) Sudden infant death syndrome (SIDS) (the sudden death of an infant in which a postmortem examination fails to confirm the cause of death): Place infants on their back to sleep. Sleeping on the side and stomach has been associated with increased rates of SIDS.

      (1) **ALERT:** The American Academy of Pediatrics recommends against co-sleeping because of its association with increased incidence of SIDS.
      (2) Peak age is 3 months; higher incidence in premature infants and during winter and spring months.
      c) Car seat: Car seats should be placed backward facing until 20 lb and 12 months. Infants weighing more than 20 lb prior to 12 months should be placed in a convertible rear and forward–facing car seat for infants greater than 20 lb.
      d) Falls
      (1) Never leave an infant alone on high surfaces.
      e) Inflicted injury
      (1) Never leave an infant alone with a pet or sibling.
      (2) Never shake a baby.

              (3) Check the temperature of formula; it should feel lukewarm when a few drops are placed on the caretaker's skin.

       f) Bath safety

              (1) Constantly hold an infant in a bath tub because of the risk of drowning.

              (2) Check temperature of the water and have no more than 2 inches of water to prevent burns and drowning.

              (3) Place the hot water heater temperature at or below 120 °F.

  2.   4 to 6 Months

     a) Falls

              (1) Baby gates should be used at the bottom and top of stairs beginning at 5 months.

     b) Aspiration and choking

              (1) Small objects should be removed from the child's reach because of the risk of aspiration as the infant puts all things in the mouth.

     c) Electrocution

              (1) Outlet covers should be put in place to avoid the risk of electrocution as the child becomes mobile.

  3.   7 to 9 Months

     a) Accidents

              (1) Remove lamps from tables as lamp cords can be pulled.

              (2) Consider removing coffee tables or padding corners to prevent injury.

              (3) With developing pincer grasp, infant places small objects in mouth; remove all potential dangers from the environment, including lint, small beans, small toy parts, and pins.

     b) Poisoning

              (1) Place cabinet locks on cabinets with poisonous chemicals and breakables.

              (2) Ensure that poisons are kept in their original container.

              (3) Place poison control number on the refrigerator to contact in the event of an accidental poisoning.

              (4) In the event of ingestion of a potentially hazardous substance, call poison control, give nothing by mouth, and avoid inducing vomiting because of potential harm to the upper gastrointestinal tract (syrup of ipecac is no longer recommended).

      4. 10 to 12 Months
- *a)* Reexamine the environment for environmental hazards.

H. Diet and nutrition

    1. 0 to 3 Months
- *a)* Breast milk or iron-fortified infant formula is the only nutritional requirement for infants in the first 6 months of life.
  - (1) Do not heat breast milk in microwave as the heat will destroy the immunoglobulins.

    2. 3-6 Months
- *a)* Teething begins. Provide comfort measures such as teething rings.
- *b)* A multivitamin with iron is often started at 6 months, but there is scientific question about its efficacy, except when the mother was anemic during pregnancy.
- *c)* Introduction of a cup can begin at 6 months.
- *d)* The child is physiologically ready for solid food introduction at 4 months as the tongue extrusion reflex disappears. The American Academy of Pediatrics, however, recommends that solid foods in the form of infant cereals not be introduced until 6 months of age because of the potential for development of food allergies later in life.

    3. 7 to 9 Months
- *a)* Provide Cheerios on high chair tray so as to promote the development of the pincer grasp and the ability to self-feed.
- *b)* Introduce new foods one at a time to identify food allergies.

    4. 10 to 12 Months
- *a)* The infant should be weaned from the bottle and breast to a cup.
- *b)* By 12 months the infant should be eating table food with the rest of the family.

    5. Nutrition guidelines
- *a)* Begin with formula or breast milk.
  - (1) Promote the advantages of breast milk, especially the presence of immunoglobulins for added immune protection.
- *b)* Give no more than 30 oz (900 ml) of milk each day.

      c)   Do not give milk other than formula or breast milk in the first 12 months of life because cow's milk is a poor source of iron, and both breast milk and formula have the essential nutrients and fat needed for growth and nutrition. Early introduction of cow's milk in place of formula or breast milk is associated with iron-deficiency anemia in infants. Adequate fat intake is needed for myelinization of the brain; therefore, skim milk and 2% milk are not appropriate during the first two years of life.

      d)   Give iron supplementation starting at age 4 months because the iron stores received before birth are beginning to be depleted.

      e)   Provide rice cereal as the first solid food, followed by any other infant single-grain cereal.

      f)   Give noncitrus fruits and vegetables.

      g)   After 6 months, give the infant foods with protein such as egg whites and meats.

      h)   Give junior foods or table food beginning at 9 months.

   6.   Feeding guidelines

      a)   Do not prop up a baby bottle; propping increases the risk of aspiration and otitis media.

      b)   Add fluoride supplements if the community water supply is insufficient.

      c)   Do not put food or cereal in a baby bottle; this discourages learning to use a spoon and greatly increases caloric intake leading to overweight and obesity.

      d)   Introduce one new food at a time; wait 4 to 7 days before introducing a new food to determine the infant's tolerance to it and potential for allergy.

      e)   Wean from breast or bottle to a cup by the first birthday.

I.   Dentition

   1.   Infants (0-6 months)

      a)   The infant's gums should be wiped with a moist washcloth once per day.

   2.   Infants (7-12 months)

      a)   The infant's teeth should be brushed after feedings with a soft-bristled toothbrush.

      b)   Avoid snacks and drinks with excess sugar.

      c)   Do not allow child to fall asleep with a bottle of juice in his/her mouth.

J. Parenting issues

    1. 0 to 9 Months

       a) Sleep and rest—The infant sleeps through the night with one to two naps per day.

       b) General care—Care should focus on meeting the infant's needs, cuddling, and talking to the infant.

       c) Common concerns—Parents are often concerned about "spoiling" the infant. Reassure parents that infants cannot be spoiled. No discipline is needed or appropriate in this age group.

    2. 10 to 12 Months

       a) Sleep and rest—The infant may give up one daytime nap. Nighttime sleeping is about 10 hours.

       b) Discipline—The infant understands the word "no." Limit setting can begin.

       c) Common concerns—Safety is a concern for infants who are increasingly mobile. The environment should be restructured to promote safety.

    3. Failure to thrive

       a) The weight of the child is below the third percentile for a period of time.

       b) This condition may be due to physical causes or from a deficiency in the parent-child relationship; may be due to organic or inorganic causes.

       c) If the problem is related to parental deprivation, the child's growth and development should improve with nurturing.

       d) Assessment

           (1) Assess for disparities among chronologic age, mental age, and bone age.

           (2) Observe for altered body posture; the child may be stiff or floppy and may not cuddle.

           (3) Assess for delayed psychosocial behavior; the child may rarely smile or talk.

           (4) Review the child's history for sleep disturbances; growth hormone is released during sleep.

           (5) Assess for inadequate feeding techniques, such as bottle propping, insufficient burping, diluting formula, or giving too much water.

           (6) Assess for degree of stimulation and parental knowledge of child development.

  e) Interventions
   (1) Rule out physiologic causes before diagnosing the condition as failure to thrive.
   (2) Teach the parents proper feeding and interactive techniques.
   (3) Help the parents recognize and respond to the child's cues.
   (4) Act as a role model for the parents.

XIII. Developmental milestones and approaches to care: Toddler (ages 1 to 3)

 A. Overview
  1. This is a period of slow growth, with a weight gain of 4 to 9 lb (2 to 4 kg) over 2 years.
  2. Vision is still not mature.
  3. The toddler requires 10 hours of sleep at night plus one daytime nap.

 B. Psychosocial development
  1. The toddler is egocentric.
  2. Separation anxiety continues to be present from late infancy; often increases in intensity through the middle of toddlerhood.
   a) The toddler sees bedtime as desertion. Sleep issues are common problems often resulting from separation anxiety. Transitional objects such as special blankets and stuffed animals may ease the transition to sleep and being alone. (Transitional objects provide security. As long as they do not interfere with daily functioning and social interactions, they are not detrimental to mental health.)
   b) The toddler develops a fear of the dark.
   c) Separation anxiety demonstrates closeness between the toddler and the parent; the toddler screams and cries when the parent leaves, then may sulk and engage in comfort measures.
   d) The parent who is leaving should say so and should promise to return.
    (1) The parent should leave a personal item with the toddler.
    (2) Prepare the parent for the toddler's reaction and explain that this process promotes trust.

3. To promote autonomy, let the toddler perform developmentally appropriate tasks independently and praise success. Examples include putting toys away when it is time to "clean up," self-feeding, and the beginning of self-dressing.

C. Cognitive development
   1. The toddler learns through sensorimotor experiences occurring through interaction with the environment.
   2. The toddler understands object permanence.
   3. The toddler engages in ritualistic behavior to master skills and decrease anxiety.
   4. The toddler exhibits magical thinking (believes that thoughts affect actions).
   5. The toddler uses symbols (understands that gestures such as waving bye-bye have meaning).
   6. Memory and learning are enhanced by experience.
   7. The toddler shows curiosity about everything but is not intentionally destructive; this curiosity can lead to aspiration or ingestion of dangerous items.
   8. The toddler engages in parallel play with playmates (playing next to one another rather than with each other).
   9. Older toddlers use play to express feelings.
   10. The toddler lacks the concept of sharing and does not understand the value of items.
   11. The toddler points to mentioned body parts and recognizes self in mirror.

D. Language/communication
   1. Language aids the toddler's perception of feelings, experiences, and memory and provides a new way to manipulate the world.
   2. By 12 months, the toddler uses five words.
   3. By 18 months, the toddler uses up to 50 words but can point to objects when asked.
   4. By age 2, the toddler uses two- to three-word phrases and comprehends many more words.
   5. At age 3, the toddler is a chatterbox, using about 11,000 words a day.
   6. The amount the toddler speaks is influenced by the amount spoken in the toddler's home.
   7. The ability to understand speech is more important than vocalization.

ALERT: The toddler should talk by age 3; if not, seek further evaluation and assess the toddler's hearing.

E. Motor skills
1. The toddler explores the environment and is usually active.
2. The toddler uses arms to balance.
3. The toddler plants feet wide apart and walks by age 15 months; if not, seek further evaluation.
    a) Feet are flat, with no arches.
    b) Provide push-pull toys to encourage walking.
4. The toddler climbs stairs at age 21 months.
5. The toddler runs and jumps by age 2 years.
6. The toddler rides a tricycle by age 3 years.

F. Communication strategies
1. The toddler understands limits and responds to consistency and limit setting.
2. The toddler responds well to positive reinforcement.

G. Developmental approaches to care
1. Care
    a) Avoid separation from parents; keep parent in child's line of vision.
    b) Toddlers are slow to warm up because of stranger anxiety. Allow time for the toddler to become acquainted with you. Talk in a friendly voice.
    c) Be flexible and realistic. Focus on the important components of your assessment.
2. Play
    a) The toddler engages in solitary play. Toddlers often play side by side, but not together.
    b) Use transitional objects for comfort and security.
    c) Promote verbal and physical stimulation.
3. Teaching
    a) The focus of teaching is the parent. Involve the child when possible, but be realistic.

H. Reactions to illness and hospitalization
1. The toddler may become unusually compliant or aggressive.
2. The toddler may regress, losing milestones previously achieved.
3. The toddler with a chronic condition may have difficulty achieving autonomy because of increased dependency on caregivers.

4. Sensorimotor experiences may be limited and/or noxious.
5. Provide for developmentally supportive nursing interventions by promoting
   a) Choices where possible
   b) Independence when possible
   c) Gross motor activities
   d) Positive sensorimotor activities

I. Anticipatory guidance and injury prevention
   1. Crib safety—When the toddler starts climbing over the crib rails, change to a bed.
   2. Car seat—The toddler should be changed to a forward-facing car seat for children >20 lb once the toddler is 1 year old and 20 lb.
   3. Falls—Place infant gates at the top and bottom of stairs to prevent falls.
   4. Accidental poisoning—Maintain vigilance with cabinet locks and keeping poisons in their original containers.
   5. Water safety
      a) Never leave the toddler alone in the bathtub; drowning can occur in as little as 1 to 2 inches of water.
      b) Keep environment free of buckets with standing water and keep toilet bowl lids in the closed position; toddlers can drown by falling in because of their large head relative to their body.
   6. Electrocution: Maintain vigilance with plastic outlet covers; curious toddlers will stick toys and other items into outlets or other openings.
   7. Fire safety and burns
      a) Put cigarette lighters and matches in secure areas out of the toddler's reach.
      b) Place pots and pans on the stove with the handles away from the edge of the stove top to prevent the toddler from reaching for handles and pulling hot liquids down on top of himself/herself.
      c) Apply devices to prevent child from playing with stove buttons.
   8. Choking/aspiration
      a) Check the size of toy parts and other objects to prevent aspiration and choking; cut food into very small pieces.
      b) The toddler has some difficulty coordinating the swallowing reflex and speaking.

J.   Diet and nutrition
1.   The toddler eats less than during infancy because of decreased appetite and growth rates.
2.   Encourage three nutritious meals and two healthy snacks per day.
3.   Portion size is 1 teaspoon per year of age for each serving (e.g., vegetable, fruit, starch, meat).
4.   Encourage socialization at mealtimes.
5.   Discourage battles over food; toddlers will eat when they are hungry.
6.   Limit mealtime to 10 to 15 minutes; toddlers cannot sit still or focus for longer.
7.   Consider allowing toddlers to cruise with snacks or meals; many toddlers cannot sit still for a formal mealtime.
8.   Avoid foods that are high in sugar or small in size (choking hazard), especially grapes, nuts, hot dogs, dried beans, and candy.
9.   The toddler feeds himself/herself; provide finger foods to promote autonomy.
10. The toddler, at age 12 months, should be changed from formula or breast milk to whole milk until at least age 2 years. Milk intake should be limited to 24 oz/day to assure intake of other nutritious foods.

 ALERT: The fat content in whole milk is necessary for children up to 2 years of age to promote myelinization of the brain.

K.   Dentition
1.   The toddler should brush his/her teeth twice daily with a nonfluoride toothpaste designed for infants and toddlers.
2.   The toddler will have 20 deciduous teeth by 3 years of age.
3.   The first dental examination should occur by 3 years of age.

L.   Parenting issues
1.   Sleep and rest
     a) The toddler requires 12 hours of sleep per day.
     b) The toddler may give up daytime napping.
     c) Sleep problems are common in toddlers and are often due to separation anxiety and fear of the dark; transitional/security objects, such as blankets and stuffed animals, can be helpful; bedtime rituals help decrease insecurity.

2. Discipline
   a) Positive reinforcement should be used for good behavior with distraction and ignoring unwanted behavior.
   b) Time out is an appropriate discipline strategy; 1 minute of time out per 1 year of age.
   c) The toddler uses "no" excessively and shows assertiveness.
   d) The toddler is curious as to how the parents will respond to "no."
   e) The toddler becomes frustrated, wants immediate gratification, and acts out of anger; the toddler may lose control; temper tantrums are common.
   f) To prevent tantrums, the parents should keep routines simple and consistent, set reasonable limits and give rationales, avoid head-on clashes, and provide choices.
   g) During a tantrum, provide a safe environment for the toddler, identify the tantrum's cause, and help the toddler regain control.
      (1) Do not reason, threaten, promise, hit, or give in.
      (2) Do not tell the toddler to wait.
      (3) Respond consistently; follow through on discipline free of anger.
   h) Overcriticizing and restricting the toddler may dampen enthusiasm and increase feelings of shame and doubt.
3. Toilet training
   a) Training depends on the toddler's emotional readiness.
      (1) The toddler acts to please others, trusts enough to give up body products, and begins autonomous behavior.
      (2) The parents must be committed to establishing a toileting pattern and must communicate well with the toddler, offering praise for success but no punishment for failure.
   b) Training also depends on the toddler's physical readiness.
      (1) The toddler's kidneys should reach adult functioning by age 2 with mature sphincter control.
      (2) The toddler feels the discomfort of wet or messy pants, identifies elimination as the cause of this discomfort, and recognizes the sensation before excretion.
      (3) The toddler removes own clothes, walks unaided, stoops and sits, talks, and imitates others.

      c) Toilet sitting begins at age 18 months, once every 2 waking hours.

        (1) Provide a pleasant mood during this time.

        (2) The toddler should use a potty seat or potty chair.

        (3) The toddler may fear being sucked into the toilet.

        (4) The toddler is curious about excretion products.

        (5) Do not refer to bowel movements as dirty or yucky.

           (a) Excrement is the toddler's first creation.

           (b) Provide alternative toys such as clay and water.

        (6) Teach the toddler hand washing and front-to-back wiping.

      d) With increased stress, the toddler may regress; toileting may have to be retaught.

      e) Introduce underpants as a badge of success and maturity.

      f) The toddler should achieve day dryness by age 18 months to 3 years and night dryness by ages 2 to 5 years.

      g) If the toddler isn't trained by age 5 years, seek further evaluation.

XIV. Developmental milestones and approaches to care: Preschool (ages 3 to 5)

  A. Overview

    1. Slow growth continues during this period.

    2. Birth length doubles by age 4.

  B. Psychosocial development

    1. The child is in Erikson's period of initiative versus guilt; the preschooler aims to accomplish and achieve.

    2. Egocentricity decreases, and awareness of others' needs increases.

      a) The child begins sharing and taking turns but continues to have difficulty with these concepts.

      b) The child attempts to please others.

    3. The child begins to develop a conscience.

      a) The preschooler is in Kohlberg's preconventional level of morality in which the child responds to rules by authority figures; this level of morality is hierarchical and involves the avoidance of "getting in trouble."

    4. The child begins to function socially.

      a) The child learns rules.

      b) Nursery school enhances the child's social development.

     5.   The child may exhibit sibling rivalry (reinforce the fact that each child is special).

     6.   The child develops fears of such things as the dark, animal noises, and new experiences.

     7.   The child may develop an imaginary playmate to help deal with fears and loneliness; this is prevalent and normal in bright, creative children.

C. Cognitive development

     1.   The child has limited perspective and focuses on one idea at a time.

     2.   The child becomes aware of racial and sexual differences.

        a)   Boys may begin to masturbate.

        b)   Begin developmentally appropriate teaching regarding sexuality.

     3.   The child develops a body image.

        a)   The parents should promote awareness of positive aspects of both sexes.

        b)   The parents should use appropriate names for body parts.

        c)   The child can draw a person.

     4.   The child begins to have a concept of causality but still exhibits magical thinking.

     5.   The child begins to have a concept of time.

        a)   The parent can explain time by referring to events.

        b)   The child begins to have a concept of "today" and "tomorrow."

     6.   The child begins to have a concept of numbers, letters, and colors.

        a)   The child may count but may not understand what the numbers mean.

        b)   The child may recognize some letters of the alphabet.

D. Language/communication

     1.   The 3-year-old uses three- to four-word sentences but has difficulty with pronouns.

     2.   The 4-year-old uses four- to five-word sentences, names colors, and counts.

     3.   The 5-year-old uses sentences of more than five words and tells long stories.

     4.   Preschoolers are concrete thinkers. Communication and explanations should provide concrete ideas and examples; preschoolers are often scared by health care lingo.

E. Motor skills
1. The child dresses and undresses self (but may not be able to tie shoes until age 5).
2. At age 3 years, the child builds a tower of more than six blocks, walks backward up and down stairs.
3. At age 4 years, the child hops and stands on one foot for up to 5 seconds, draws a person with two to four body parts, throws overhand, and catches a ball.
4. At 5 years, the child undresses and dresses self well, runs, jumps, skips, hops, and does somersaults.
5. Child develops hand dominance.

F. Developmental approaches to care
1. Care
   a) Respect the child's privacy and modesty.
   b) Promote cooperation.
   c) Provide explanations.
2. Play
   a) The child exhibits parallel play, associative play, group play in activities with few or no rules, and independent play associated with sharing or talking.
      (1) Allow the child to handle and play with medical equipment to increase comfort level, i.e., stethoscope and BP cuff.
      (2) Engage the child in his/her favorite activities.
   b) The child engages in imaginary play (i.e., make-believe).
   c) Examples of appropriate toys include dolls, sandbox, water, blocks, crayons, clay, and finger paint.
3. Teaching
   a) The parent is the primary focus of teaching.
   b) Involve the preschooler in teaching through the use of short, simple explanations.

G. Reactions to illness and hospitalization
1. Observe for maladaptive responses to illness and hospitalization.
   a) The child shows anxiety about health care treatments and life events.
   b) The child shows fear concerning body integrity.
2. Provide for developmentally supportive nursing interventions.
   a) Use doll play to help the child prepare for or adjust to treatment.
   b) Provide adhesive bandages for cuts, because the child fears losing blood.

H. Anticipatory guidance and injury prevention
  1. Drowning
    a) Observe the preschooler near water.
    b) Use flotation devices while swimming.
    c) Lock gates surrounding swimming pools.
  2. Fire safety and burns
    a) Place matches and cigarette lighters out of reach of preschoolers.
  3. Sports safety
    a) Wear helmets while riding tricycles, scooters, and roller skating.
  4. Automobile safety
    a) The preschooler should ride in the backseat in a forward-facing car seat until 4 years and 40 lb.
    b) The preschooler should move to a booster seat at 40 lb and 4 years.

J. Diet and nutrition
  1. Encourage three nutritious meals plus two healthy snacks per day.
  2. Food jags and strong food preferences are common.
    a) Encourage parents to offer a variety of foods.
    b) Avoid battles over foods.
    c) Children often do not like food mixed together; keep foods separate.
  3. Portion size is 1 tablespoon per year of age for each serving (e.g., vegetable, fruit, starch, meat).
  4. Children establish eating behaviors (washing hands before meals, table manners, eating while seated).

K. Dentition
  1. Brush teeth twice daily and introduce dental flossing daily.
  2. Child should have an annual dental visit.

L. Parenting issues
  1. Bedwetting (enuresis)
    a) Bedwetting is a common concern in this age group. Nighttime dryness is generally achieved by age 5.
    b) Limit fluids after dinner time.
    c) Encourage toilet time prior to sleep.

ALERT: Bedwetting that is a new occurrence in a previously toilet-trained child should be discussed with the child's primary care provider. Bedwetting can be a sign of urinary tract infection, as well as other disease conditions and psychosomatic problems.

2. Discipline
   a) Disciplinary actions should be consistent; "time out" is an effective disciplinary action. Because the child has a poor concept of time, make sure the child is told when the time out is over.
   b) Do not compare one child to another in terms of abilities or psychosocial traits.

M. Readiness for kindergarten
   1. The child picks up after self.
   2. The child gets along without either parent for short periods.
   3. The child is less afraid.
   4. The child listens and follows directions.
   5. The child speaks in correct, complete sentences.

XV. Developmental milestones and approaches to care: School-age child (ages 6 to 12)

A. Overview
   1. School shapes the child's cognitive and social development.

B. Psychosocial development
   1. The school-age child is in Erikson's stage of industry versus inferiority; school is seen as the "job" of the school-age child.
   2. The teacher, perhaps the first important adult in the child's life besides the parents, may be a major influence.
   3. The child plays with peers.
      a) The child develops a first true friendship.
      b) The child develops a sense of belonging, cooperation, and compromise.
   4. The child participates in group activities, including team sports.
      a) Groups offer a testing ground for the child's interpersonal interactions, development of self-concept, and sex-role behaviors.
         (1) Groups encourage competition through fair play.
         (2) Groups relieve the child of having to make decisions.
         (3) The child's play involves group goals with interaction and cooperation.
   5. The child develops a sense of morality (the conventional stage of Kohlberg), in which the child conforms to social norms and customs.
      a) The early school-age child sees actions as either right or wrong.

b) After age 9, the child understands intent and differing points of view.

c) The child plays by the rules but often cheats.

6. The child compares own body to others' and may become modest.

7. The child participates in family activities.

8. The child becomes aware of social roles.

9. The child engages in fantasy play and daydreaming.

10. The child may exhibit a fear of death and school phobias; these fears may cause psychosomatic illness.

11. The child likes to accomplish tasks.

C. Cognitive development

1. The child enters Piaget's cognitive level of concrete operations.

a) The child develops a sense of time and space, cause and effect, nesting (building blocks, puzzle pieces), reversibility, conservation (permanence of mass and volume), and numbers.

2. The child understands the relationship of parts to the whole (fractions).

3. The child learns to classify objects in more than one way.

4. The child becomes interested in board games, cards, and collections.

5. The child learns to read and spell.

D. Physical development/motor skills

1. Slow growth continues during this period; height increases about 2.5 in. a year and weight doubles between ages 6 and 12.

2. Both sexes are about the same size until approximately age 9, when some females begin puberty and grow faster. (Precocious puberty is when breast development begins before age 7 in White females and before age 6 in African American females.)

3. Bones grow faster than muscles and ligaments; therefore, the child is limber and prone to bone fractures.

4. Large and small muscle groups are refined.

5. Lymphoid tissue hypertrophies to maximum size.

6. Vision matures by age 6.

a) Annual visual acuity is tested using a wall chart (Snellen or Lea) or a Titmus machine.

b) Common signs of visual acuity problems include the child having trouble seeing the blackboard in school (moving to sit in the front row) or having trouble seeing the television set (moving to sit near the television).

E. Communication
   1. Language development is perfected.
F. Developmental approaches to care
   1. Care
      a) Involve the child in care; assent is recommended for treatments and for research.
      b) Explain procedures, equipment, and care.
      c) Provide time for interviewing the child separately from the parent.
   2. Play
      a) Inquire about favorite activities.
      b) Promote peer contact where possible.
   3. Teaching
      a) Parents and schools share the responsibility for health teaching, with parents being the primary providers of information and values.
      b) Provide explanations and answer questions in an age-appropriate manner.
G. Reactions to illness and hospitalization
   1. Observe for maladaptive responses to illness and hospitalization.
      a) The child exhibits signs of isolation because of school absenteeism, lack of peer contact, and increased dependence on caregivers.
      b) The young school-age child still exhibits magical thinking, believing that disease and hospitalization are punishment.
   2. Provide for developmentally supportive nursing interventions:
      a) Promote school attendance.
      b) Educate the child about his/her illness and reinforce that illness is not his/her fault.
      c) Collaborate with the school nurse and teachers regarding the child's abilities and needs.
      d) Encourage participation in activities and care as much as possible.
H. Anticipatory guidance and injury prevention

ALERT: Accidents are a major cause of death and disability among school-age children.

1. Sports safety: Teach children to wear helmets at all times when bicycling, skateboarding, roller-skating, rollerblading, and so on.
2. Automobile safety
    a) In many states, booster seats are required for children age 4 (>40 lb) to 8 years and 80 lb.
    b) The back seat is recommended for all children 12 years and under.
3. Water safety: Supervise children near water. Teach children to stay away from fast-moving water and to always enter water feet first.
4. Stranger safety: Discuss importance of not getting into car with a stranger; consider a code word that only parents and child know for use by anyone with whom the child would be transported.
5. Firearm safety
    a) Avoid having firearms in the home.
    b) Lock ammunition and firearms in separate cabinets.
    c) Talk about what to do if child finds a firearm at school or a friend's house ("Stop, Don't Touch, Run Away, Tell an Adult").

 ALERT: School-age children are open to role play. This is an excellent way to discuss potential hazards and to teach ways of addressing them. Role play provides a real-life way of practicing one's response.

I. Diet and nutrition
    1. The school-age period is one in which the child is greatly influenced by peers and the media regarding diet and nutrition.
    2. This is a time when healthy diet and activity habits are established.
        a) Encourage three nutritious meals and two healthy snacks per day.
        b) Discuss healthy lifestyle choices regarding food choices and physical activity; limit television-watching time.
    3. Overweight puts children at risk for type 2 diabetes, hypertension, and hyperlipidemia.
        a) Monitor BMI with yearly growth chart documentation and assessment.
        b) Refer for nutrition consultation and medical evaluation for BMI >85%.

J. Dentition
1. The first primary tooth is displaced by a permanent tooth at age 6 to 7, and permanent teeth replace primary teeth at a rate of 4 per year until age 12; by age 12, all permanent teeth are present except the final molars; the jaw grows to accommodate the permanent teeth.
2. Dental visits are annual.
3. Brush teeth twice daily with a fluoride toothpaste, and floss daily.
4. This is a prime time for the development of dental caries; nutrition and dental education should be reinforced in the home and in the school.

K. Parenting issues
1. Communication: The school-age child develops increased independence from parents with wider influences of peers and teachers.
   a) Encourage independence while increasing personal responsibilities.
   b) Use active listening.
   c) Become involved in the child's activities outside of school.
2. Discipline
   a) Use praise and support.
   b) Discuss consequences of actions.
   c) Discuss conflict resolution among peer group.

XVI. Developmental milestones and approaches to care: Adolescent (ages 13 to 18)

A. Overview
1. Adolescence is a rapid growth period characterized by puberty-related changes in body structure and psychosocial adjustment.

B. Psychosocial development
1. Adolescents experience Erikson's psychosocial stage of identity versus role confusion. This is also a time in which the adolescent struggles to confront issues of morality, sexuality, and future occupation.
2. Early adolescence is spent coping with changes in the physical self and becoming aware of the bodies of others.
   a) Fantasy thoughts and daydreams allow the adolescent to role-play different social situations.

   b) Suggest that the adolescent keep a diary to express feelings.
  3. Middle adolescence involves exploring and identifying one's values and defining oneself.
   a) Peers may influence fad behaviors, values, or conformity.
   b) Interest in the opposite sex increases; some adolescents may experience same-sex attractions.
  4. Late adolescence involves maturation, expressed by independence from parents and participation in society.
   a) The adolescent begins to plan for the future.
  5. Adolescence ends when the youth is physically and financially independent of parents.

C. Cognitive development
  1. The adolescent develops abstract thinking and an increased ability to analyze, synthesize, and use logic.
  2. The adolescent reaches the cognitive level of an adult.

D. Development of secondary sex characteristics
  1. Development in the female
   a) The hypothalamus signals the pituitary to release gonadotropins.
    (1) This increases the secretion of luteinizing hormone (LH) and follicle-stimulating hormone (FSH), which stimulate ovarian development and estrogen production.
    (2) Estrogen produces all secondary sex characteristics except axillary and pubic hair, which are controlled by adrenal androgens.
   b) Breast development (thelarche), the first sign of puberty (as per the Tanner assessment), begins on average at age 10 with the bud stage (range = 7-13 years).
    (1) Breast development takes approximately 3 years to complete.
    (2) Breast development ends shortly after the first menses.
   c) Fatty tissue in the thighs, hips, and breast increases; the hips broaden.
   d) Pubic hair appears on average at age 11 and increases with the progression of puberty and for several years after puberty.
   e) The onset of menses occurs between ages 8 and 16, or approximately 3 years after breast development begins; menses initially may be irregular.

      f)   The growth spurt begins early in puberty, shortly after breast budding, before menarche. Females grow up to 3 in. (8 cm)/year, stopping growth around age 16. Compared with males, females have a shorter period of time in which to grow and a lower rate of growth during the pubertal growth spurt.

      g)   The sweat glands and sebaceous glands become more active; body odor and acne increase.

2.   Development in the male

    a)   The hypothalamus signals the pituitary gonadotropins to release LH and FSH.

        (1) LH results in testicular enlargement and the development of Leydig's cells in the testes, which produce testosterone.

        (2) FSH stimulates the development of the seminiferous tubules of the testes, leading to spermatogenesis and fertility.

    b)   Testicular enlargement signals the start of puberty (as per the Tanner assessment), beginning approximately at 11 years, with a range of 10 to 15 years.

        (1) The scrotum enlarges, and the penis elongates and widens.

        (2) The penis reaches adult size at about age 17.

    c)   Muscle mass increases, the chest broadens, facial and body hair proliferates, and laryngeal cartilage growth deepens the voice.

    d)   Pubic hair growth begins on average at 12 years and continues to grow and increase until approximately age 20.

    e)   The male's height spurt begins 2 years later than the female's.

        (1) The male can grow up to 3.5 in. (9 cm)/year, with growth ending around age 20.

        (2) Compared with females, males have a longer period of time in which to grow and have a higher rate of growth during the pubertal growth spurt.

    f)   The sweat glands and sebaceous glands become more active; body odor and acne increase.

    g)   Nocturnal emissions ("wet dreams") are common.

    h)   Masturbation is common.

E. High-risk behaviors
  1. Motor vehicle accidents are the primary cause of mortality and morbidity; car safety information is essential in this age.
  2. Suicide is the third leading cause of death among middle and late adolescents (homicide is second).
    a) Assess body image and self-concept.
    b) Discuss peer relationships and social support.
  3. More than 46% of all adolescents have had sexual intercourse by high-school graduation.
    a) Sex education must be provided for both adolescents and their parents; communication between them should be encouraged.
    b) Sex education must include anatomy and physiology, as well as values clarification, communication skills, role play and role modeling, alternatives, and the concept of personal responsibility and respect for others.
  4. Smoking and drug and alcohol abuse are common risk-taking behaviors of adolescents; others include use of anabolic steroids and inhalants, tanning, and gambling.
    a) Cognitive and affective information is needed.
    b) Seeing the effects of drunk driving and hearing the stories of addicted persons can be effective in decreasing these behaviors.

F. Communication strategies
  1. Use active listening techniques.
  2. Use open-ended questions in patient interview rather than yes/no questions.
  3. Remain nonjudgmental; focus on obtaining health-related information and identifying risk factors to guide teaching and care.
  4. Do not promise to keep information confidential if it involves potential danger to the youth by himself/herself or by others, or danger to others, especially if sharing information is required by law.

G. Developmental approaches to care
  1. Care
    a) Provide privacy and respect modesty.
    b) Interview separately from parent.
  2. Play
    a) Encourage peer interaction.

3. Teaching
    a) Teaching should involve the parent in the majority of situations.
    b) Focus on responsibility and understanding of health-related issues.

H. Reactions to illness and hospitalization
    1. Observe for maladaptive responses to illness and hospitalization.
        a) Personality and sexual identity may be hampered.
        b) Establishment of independence may be difficult.
        c) Establishment of peer and sexual relationships may be difficult.
    2. Provide for developmentally supportive nursing interventions.
        a) Promote normalcy; reinforce normal findings.
        b) Promote peer interaction.
        c) Promote independence and self-care.
        d) Respect and maintain privacy.
        e) Provide emotional support.

I. Anticipatory guidance and injury prevention
    1. Assess weight and height for potential for anorexia, bulimia, and overweight.
        a) Consider type 2 diabetes as a potential result of overweight.
        b) Remember that bulimia may be present in children who are of normal weight.
        c) When assessing for the potential for eating disorders, assess the adolescent's sense of body image and identity.
    2. Perform a sexual history.
        a) Assess for risk factors for pregnancy; discuss contraception and alternatives as appropriate.
        b) Assess for heterosexual, homosexual, and bisexual behavior; be careful not to assume gender of sexual partner(s).
            (1) Provide education regarding sexually transmitted diseases.
    3. Assess for risk factors for substance abuse and provide education as necessary.
        a) Use the HEADS assessment to assess Adolescent Risk Profile
            (1) Ask about *H*ome, *E*ducation, *A*ctivities, *D*rugs, *S*exual activity/identity, Suicide/depression.

J. Diet and nutrition
1. Nutritional needs greatly increase during this period of rapid growth and development.
2. Dietary intake is often unhealthy or inadequate for growth and development.
3. Eating is a social event and is influenced by peers.
4. The adolescent may diet excessively to attain a desirable body image.

K. Dentition
1. Dental appointments should be annual.
2. Brush teeth twice daily and floss daily.
3. Final molars (wisdom teeth) may erupt

L. Parenting issues
1. Communication
   a) Limit setting is successful when it is understood and not arbitrary.
   b) Give freedom and choices where possible.
2. Discipline
   a) Focus on encouraging the adolescent to make decisions and understand consequences.
   b) Save battles for the important things.

CHAPTER
4

Genetic Alterations

LEARNING OBJECTIVE

1. Determine the risk of transmission of autosomal dominant, autosomal recessive, and sex-linked conditions.

I. Introduction

A. Human cells contain 46 chromosomes in each nucleus (23 pairs).
   1. Each chromosome contains thousands of genes.
   2. Chromosomes are shaped like an X (except the male Y).

B. Genes are the structures responsible for hereditary characteristics; they may or may not be expressed or passed to the next generation.

C. *Genotype* refers to the sequence and combination of genes on a chromosome.

D. Alleles are pairs of genes located on the same site on paired chromosomes
   1. *Homozygous alleles* are identical (DD or dd).
   2. *Heterozygous alleles* are two different alleles for the same trait (Dd).

E. Mendel's law states that one gene for each hereditary property is received from each parent; one is dominant (expressed) and one is recessive.

F. A *karyotype* is the chromosomal pattern of a cell, including genotype, number of chromosomes, and normality or abnormality of the chromosomes.

G. A *phenotype* is the observable expression of the genes (e.g., hair and eye color, body build, allergies).

H. Congenital means present at birth because of abnormal development in utero (teratology).
   1. Some genetic disorders may be noticeable at birth, and some may not appear for decades.

II. Altered cell division

A. *Mitosis* is normal cell division, resulting in an exact copy of the parent cell.

B. *Meiosis* is normal cell division of the ova and spermatozoon for procreation, resulting in 23 chromosomes (one chromosome from each of the 23 pairs); this is called reduction division.

C. *Mutation* is a spontaneous alteration in genes or chromosomes not present in the previous generation.

D. *Nondisjunction* is the failure of one pair of chromosomes from either parent to separate during meiosis, usually resulting in 45 or 47 chromosomes in the offspring (trisomy indicates 47).

E. *Translocation* occurs when the chromosome breaks; the parts may connect to another chromosome, or the genes may switch their order or spacing.

F. *Mosaicism* refers to a different number of chromosomes in different organs of the body or a combination of the above alterations.

III. Autosomal diseases and disorders

A. Autosomal chromosomes represent the first 22 pairs.

B. In *dominant disorders*, only one defective gene or set of genes is passed by one parent.
   1. Examples include Huntington disease, osteogenesis imperfecta, neurofibromatosis, and night blindness.
   2. Offer genetic counseling: *with each pregnancy in which only one parent is a heterozygotic carrier comes a 50% chance of having a child with the disease or disorder and a 50% chance of having a normal child.*

		Parent with normal genes (DD)	
		D	D
Parent with affected genes (Dd)	D	DD	DD
	d	Dd	Dd

DD is normal; Dd has the condition

C. In *recessive disorders*, both parents must pass the defective gene or set of genes to the child
   1. Almost all carriers are free of symptoms; a carrier has one healthy chromosome and one affected chromosome.
   2. Examples include cystic fibrosis, sickle cell anemia, phenylketonuria (PKU), Tay-Sachs disease, and albinism.
   3. Offer genetic counseling: *with each pregnancy in which each parent is a heterozygous carrier comes a 25% chance of having a child with the disease or disorder, a 50% chance of having a child who is a carrier, and a 25% chance of having a normal child.*

		Parent with affected genes (Dd)	
		D	d
Parent with affected genes (Dd)	D	DD	Dd
	d	Dd	dd

(DD is normal; Dd is a carrier; dd has the condition)

IV. Genetic sex-linked (X-linked) recessive diseases and disorders

A. These are associated with the 23rd pair of chromosomes.

B. Sex-linked genetic disorders are carried on the X chromosome and passed by women; women do not usually get these disorders because their other healthy X chromosome will predominate (men have no other X chromosome to oppose the affected X; the Y chromosome is usually small).

C. Examples include hemophilia, color blindness, one type of muscular dystrophy, and glucose-6-phosphate dehydrogenase (G-6-PD) deficiency.

D. Offer genetic counseling; *the father with a sex-linked disorder will pass the trait to all of his daughters but none of his sons; however, none of his children will have the disease; his daughters will have a 50% chance with each pregnancy of passing the disease or disorder to their sons.*

V. Chromosomal disorders/syndromes

A syndrome is a recognizable pattern of characteristics resulting from a common cause or appearing together to present a clinical picture of a disease or chronic condition.

A. Down syndrome (trisomy 21)
  1. Down syndrome is usually related to nondisjunction, with 3 chromosomes on the 21st pair (total of 47 chromosomes); the risk of nondisjunction increases with increasing maternal age.
  2. Assessment findings include a small head with slow brain growth, upward slanting palpebral fissures (the opening between the eyelids), Brushfield's spots (marbling and speckling of the iris), a broad flat nose and low-set ears, a protruding tongue (because of a small oral cavity), short stature with pudgy hands, a transverse palmar/simian crease (a single crease across the palm), hypotonia, and mild to moderate retardation.

      3.   The child faces an increased risk of associated problems, such as congenital heart defects, strabismus, chronic myelogenous leukemia, and a weaker immune response to infection.

      4.   No specific treatment exists beyond ordinary care for the individual with cognitive delays.

B. Turner syndrome (occurs only in females)

      1.   The child has an XO karyotype for the 23rd chromosome (monosomy = loss of one chromosome) (O represents the failure to receive one X chromosome from one parent) with only 45 chromosomes—no Barr body (the inactive X on the 23rd pair).

      2.   Assessment findings include short stature, webbing of the neck (extra skin from the ear to the shoulder), a low posterior hairline, low-set ears, gonadal-ovarian dysgenesis, and the lack of sexual development or menses at puberty.

      3.   The child is learning disabled and may have difficulty in social situations.

      4.   The child has associated cardiac and renal abnormalities.

      5.   The child is treated with estrogen to develop secondary sex characteristics and menses but remains sterile.

C. Klinefelter syndrome (occurs only in males)

      1.   The child has an extra chromosome on the 23rd pair, resulting in an XXY karyotype (47 chromosomes).

      2.   Assessment findings include a tall, thin body (until the estrogen level stimulates increased body fat distribution, especially gynecomastia) and the failure of secondary sex characteristics to develop at puberty.

      3.   The child is learning disabled.

      4.   The child is treated with androgens but remains sterile.

CHAPTER
5

Hematologic Conditions

LEARNING OBJECTIVES

After studying this chapter, you should be able to:

1. Describe the impact of bone marrow failure.

2. Discuss conditions associated with alterations in red blood cell and platelet functioning.

3. Plan appropriate nursing care for pediatric patients with anemia and clotting deficiencies.

I. Chapter overview

Knowledge of the anatomy and physiology of blood and its components provides the foundation for understanding the conditions associated with altered hematologic function. Hematologic conditions can be approached from the perspective of the ways in which they affect normal functioning of red blood cells and clotting. Assessment and nursing interventions are geared toward preventing and controlling the problems associated with the alteration and promoting normal function.

II. Introduction: Composition and function of blood

A. Blood composition
1. Formed elements (cells): erythrocytes (red blood cells or RBCs), thrombocytes (platelets or PLTs), and five types of leukocytes (white blood cells or WBCs)—neutrophils (immature band neutrophils called "bands" and mature segmented neutrophils called "segs"), lymphocytes, monocytes, eosinophils, and basophils
   a) All blood cells are formed in the bone marrow originating from the hematopoietic stem cell.
   b) Early in utero, all blood cells are made by the liver and spleen; these organs retain their ability to make blood cells throughout life.
   c) Before birth, the bone marrow becomes the main producer of blood cells.
2. Plasma
   a) Approximately 90% of plasma is composed of water.
   b) Approximately 10% of plasma is solutes such as electrolytes, proteins, dissolved nutrients, clotting factors, anticoagulants, and antibodies.
B. Functions of blood
1. Blood cells and plasma play a major role in the following:
   a) Oxygenation of body tissues
   b) Cellular nutrition
   c) Excretion via transport of wastes to other organs
   d) Maintenance of acid-base balance
   e) Regulation of body temperature
   f) Defense against foreign antigens
   g) Transport of hormones

C. Red blood cell functioning: An overview
1. RBCs carry oxygenated hemoglobin from the lung to the tissues of the body and deoxygenated hemoglobin from the tissues to the lungs.
2. RBC production is stimulated by two mechanisms that stimulate the bone marrow:
    a) Tissue hypoxia
    b) Renal production of erythropoietin (which is stimulated by hypoxia)
    c) It is important to know that the driving factor in RBC release from the bone marrow is the ability of the tissues' need for oxygen rather than the number of RBCs circulating.
3. Normal RBCs live 120 days.
    a) When an RBC dies or is destroyed (hemolysis), most of the iron is conserved.
    b) Unconjugated bilirubin (also called indirect bilirubin) is one of the byproducts of RBC hemolysis.
    c) Byproducts of the breakdown of RBCs include iron and bilirubin. Iron is reabsorbed and reused. Bilirubin, in its unconjugated (also called indirect) form, is present in the systemic circulation for transport to the liver. In the liver it is conjugated and becomes conjugated (also called direct) bilirubin that is removed from the body through the bile and ultimately through the stool.
    d) Liver enzymes convert unconjugated bilirubin into conjugated bilirubin (also called direct) in the liver for excretion in the bile.
4. Reticulocytes are immature RBCs that comprise 0.5% to 1.5% of the total RBCs circulating. They are an indicator of hematopoiesis (formation of blood) from the bone marrow.
    a) An increase in reticulocytes indicates an increased rate of production of RBCs from the bone marrow, whereas a decreased number of reticulocytes in the blood indicates a decreased production of RBCs from the bone marrow as seen in bone marrow suppression.
5. Excess RBC production is called polycythemia; it results in increased blood viscosity.
6. The newborn normally has a high RBC count (4.8 to 7.1 million/mm^3).
    a) A normal RBC count is 4.5 to 5.5 million/mm^3.

7. RBC characteristics

   a) RBCs are described using laboratory values called RBC indices. These RBC indices describe size (macro-, micro-, and normocytic) and hemoglobin content of the RBC that affects its color (hyper-, hypo-, and normochromic).

   (1) Mean corpuscular volume (MCV)

   (a) MCV indicates the average size of the RBC.

   (b) Normocytic cells (normal size) are indicated by an MCV value between 75 and 94 mm^3 with variability based on age and gender.

   (c) Macrocytic cells (large size) are indicated by an MCV >94 mm^3; clinical implications include folate or vitamin B$_{12}$ deficiency, aplastic anemia, immune hemolytic anemia.

   (d) Microcytic cells (small size) are indicated by an MCV <75 mm^3; clinical implications include iron deficiency anemia, lead poisoning, thalassemia.

   (2) Mean corpuscular hemoglobin (MCH)

   (a) MCH indicates the average weight of hemoglobin per RBC.

   (b) Normal MCH values for the child are 25 to 33 picograms (pg)/cell.

   (c) Clinical implications for increases and decreases in MCH are the same as for MCV.

   (3) Mean corpuscular hemoglobin concentration (MCHC)

   (a) MCHC indicates the average concentration of hemoglobin per RBC

   (b) Normochromic cells containing a normal amount of hemoglobin (Hgb) are indicated by an MCHC of 33% to 36% Hgb/dl with variability based on age.

   (c) Hyperchromic cells containing an increased amount of hemoglobin are indicated by an MCHC of >36% Hgb/dl with variability based on age.

   i) Clinical implications for an increased MCHC include hereditary spherocytosis.

        (*d*) Hypochromic cells containing a decreased amount of hemoglobin are indicated by an MCHC of <33% Hgb/dl.

            i) Clinical implications for a decreased MCHC include iron deficiency and thalassemia.

    (4) Red cell distribution width (RDW)

        (*a*) RDW indicates the uniformity of RBC size.

        (*b*) Normal RDW values for the child are 11.5 to 14.5.

        (*c*) Anisocytosis (increased RDW) indicates greater cell size variability.

            i) Clinical implications for an increased RDW include iron deficiency anemia, folic acid deficiency anemia, and vitamin B_{12} deficiency anemia.

8. RBC hemolysis

    a) There are a variety of conditions that can result in RBC hemolysis, including sickle cell disease, hereditary spherocytosis, hemolytic disease of the newborn, blood transfusion reaction, and others.

D. Hemoglobin functioning: An overview

    1. Hemoglobin is the component of the RBC that carries oxygen and delivers it to the tissue of the body.

    2. Hemoglobin contains iron, which gives hemoglobin its pigment.

    3. Hemoglobin is made up of two different pairs of globin molecules. The type of globin molecules depends on the stage in life and any abnormalities of the genes that regulate hemoglobin formation.

        a) Hemoglobin F: This is the type of hemoglobin made during fetal life. It absorbs oxygen at a lower tension; at birth, 75% of hemoglobin is HbF.

        b) Hemoglobin A: This type of hemoglobin is made in postnatal life and slowly replaces HbF during the first year of life. It is composed of 2 α and 2 β globin chains.

        (1) The lowest point of HbA and HbF is 4 to 6 months of age, which is when iron should be added to the diet.

4. Normal hemoglobin levels in the child are 11.5 to 14.5 g/dl with variability based on age and gender. Anemia is the term used to describe a low hemoglobin count.

5. Clinical implications for an increase in the hemoglobin level include situations in which there are more cells or less fluid, such as polycythemia vera, congenital heart disease, chronic hypoxia, high altitudes, and fluid loss (dehydration).

6. Clinical implications for a decrease in the hemoglobin level include situations in which there are fewer cells or more fluid, such as aplastic anemia, renal disease, iron deficiency, bone marrow suppression, sickle cell disease, hereditary spherocytosis, hemorrhage, and fluid volume overload.

E. Hematocrit overview

1. Hematocrit is the percentage of packed RBCs to whole blood.

2. Hematocrit expresses the relationship of cells to fluid.

3. Hematocrit exists in a constant relationship to hemoglobin, which is three times the hemoglobin concentration.

    a) The hematocrit level rises and falls in the same direction and for the same reasons as does the hemoglobin level.

4. Normal hematocrit levels for the child are 35% to 45% with variability based on age and gender.

5. Clinical implications for increases and decreases in hematocrit are the same as for hemoglobin.

III. Conditions affecting the red blood cell

A. Anemia

1. Overview

    a) Anemia is defined as a decrease in the amount of serum hemoglobin.

    b) Anemia constitutes a symptom rather than a diagnosis.

    c) It is classified according to morphology (RBC characteristics) and etiology.

    d) Anemia can be either acute or chronic.

2. Etiology

    a) Anemia may result from a decrease in production, size, or lifespan of RBCs or from a reduction in the amount of hemoglobin.

    b) Causes of anemia can be categorized in the following ways:

        (1) Nutritional deficiencies

        (2) Increased hemolysis (RBC destruction).

              (3) Impaired or decreased rate of production by the bone marrow or due to decreased erythropoietin release from the kidneys

              (4) Excessive blood loss (acute or chronic).

3. Clinical manifestations

    a) Anemia can be either acute or chronic.

              (1) Chronic anemia: Overall, chronic anemia is well tolerated by the body because of the body's compensatory mechanisms. Clinical manifestations include growth retardation, delayed sexual maturation, increased heart rate and cardiac output, and cardiac murmur.

              (2) Acute anemia: Clinical manifestations of acute anemia are typically a result of acute tissue hypoxia. These clinical manifestations include muscle weakness, fatigue, pallor, headache, lightheadedness, increased heart rate, increased cardiac output, and heart murmur.

4. Assessment

    a) Take the child's diet history; document the nutrients needed to make RBCs (iron, folic acid, vitamin B_{12}).

    b) Note malnutrition or anorexia.

    c) Check for medications that interfere with RBC production, such as phenytoin (Dilantin) and sulfonamides.

    d) Check urine, stool, and emesis for blood.

    e) Assess skin color for pallor from tissue hypoxia.

    f) Check hemoglobin and RBC levels.

    g) Note skin breakdown from poor tissue oxygenation.

    h) Check for jaundice and pruritus from large amounts of unconjugated bilirubin in the blood related to hemolysis of the RBCs; check bilirubin level.

    i) Note increased pulse and respiratory rates as the body compensates for hypoxia.

    j) Note altered neurologic status or behavioral changes from poor oxygenation to the brain.

    k) Assess for hepatomegaly and splenomegaly from sequestered RBCs related to the hematopoietic and phagocytic functions of the liver and spleen.

    l) Note weakness or low exercise tolerance.

    m) Note growth retardation or failure to achieve developmental milestones.

5. Interventions
   a) Determine and eliminate the causes of anemia.
   b) Decrease oxygen demands for acute anemia: plan activities, provide passive stimulation, allow frequent rest, give small frequent feedings with softer foods, elevate the head of the bed.
   c) Implement proper hand washing and mouth care.
   d) Maintain the child's normal body temperature.

B. Iron deficiency anemia
   1. Overview
      a) Iron deficiency anemia is one of the most prevalent nutritional disorders in the United States.
      b) Iron is a necessary component of normal hemoglobin formation. When iron is insufficient, the hemoglobin concentration in the RBC is low, causing RBCs to be microcytic (small) and insufficient for carrying oxygen.
   2. Etiology
      a) Common causes of iron deficiency anemia
         (1) Inadequate dietary intake: Excessive whole milk intake in a child over 12 months of age is a common causative factor. Whole milk does not contain sufficient iron, such as found in iron-fortified cereals and formula.
         (2) Impaired absorption of iron
         (3) Blood loss
         (4) Excessive demands for iron required for growth
      b) Risk factors
         (1) Premature infants
            (*a*) Anemia is secondary to decreased fetal iron supply because the iron is transferred from the mother to the fetus at the fastest rate in the last trimester of pregnancy.
         (2) Infants of a multiple pregnancy (twins/triplets).
            (*a*) Anemia results from this risk factor because of the sharing of iron from the maternal iron source during pregnancy.
         (3) Low-income children 6 to 24 months
            (*a*) There is a decreased prevalence of anemia because of the federal Women, Infants, and Children (WIC) program.

(4) Adolescents
  (a) Anemia is secondary to an adolescent's increased growth rate accompanied by poor eating habits.

3. Assessment
  a) Complete a dietary history and history of present illness.
  b) Assess for signs of acute anemia such as tachycardia, pallor, and lethargy.
  c) Obtain blood for complete blood cell count (use heel stick for infants).

4. Interventions
  a) Provide short-term iron supplementation to correct the acute anemia and long-term dietary modification to include foods rich in iron.
  b) Perform dietary teaching regarding iron-rich foods as indicated.
  c) Administer iron supplementation as necessary.
    (1) Iron temporarily stains teeth. Use a dropper at the back of the mouth.
    (2) Iron is best absorbed between meals and with a citrus fruit or juice.
      (a) Antacids, tetracycline, and histamine H_2 receptor blockers may interfere with absorption of iron.
    (3) Stools should be a dark black or tarry green when iron levels are adequate.
    (4) Place iron out of the reach of children because of the risk of iron overdose and toxicity.
    (5) Brush teeth after administration of iron.

C. Aplastic anemia
  1. Overview
    a) Aplastic anemia results from the bone marrow's failure to produce RBCs and other blood components.
  2. Etiology
    a) A congenital or acquired condition, it is commonly caused by an autoimmune process or certain medications, radiation, and benzene products, although 50% of cases are idiopathic.
  3. Assessment
    a) Prepare for and assist with bone marrow aspiration in the iliac crest. (The diagnosis is confirmed by abnormal findings.)

        b)   Assess for symptoms of anemia, platelet deficiency, and WBC deficiency.

4.   Interventions

     a)   Provide transfusion support.

     b)   Administer immunosuppressive medications (e.g., cortisone, cyclosporine) to stop the autoimmune process.

     c)   Prepare for possible bone marrow transplantation as a curative measure.

     d)   Treatment is similar to that for leukemia.

     e)   If platelets and white blood cells are also affected, initiate interventions for hemostasis and decreased immunity.

D. Hereditary spherocytosis

1.   Overview

     a)   Hereditary spherocytosis (HS) is an abnormal fragility and inflexibility of the RBC membrane. The spherocyte is spherical (instead of biconcave) and cannot change its shape as needed to fit through the vessels. These RBCs are susceptible to trapping in the microvasculature and chronic hemolysis (breakdown) as the spleen traps and destroys RBCs (hemolysis).

2.   Etiology

     a)   HS is caused by an autosomal dominant gene that affects the RBC membrane (called a spherocyte).

     b)   Although the defect causes clinical manifestations that mimic the RBC rigidity and susceptibility to hemolysis, as in sickle cell disease, HS is not caused by a defect in the hemoglobin.

3.   Clinical manifestations

     a)   Symptoms of intermittent acute and ongoing chronic anemia are present.

     b)   Early RBC destruction secondary to RBC fragility (i.e., increased hemolysis) leads to:

        (1)   Chronic anemia (usually hemoglobin is 7 to 10 g/dl)

        (2)   Jaundice (most commonly scleral icterus) caused by increased hemolysis

        (3)   Splenomegaly (because of RBC trapping in the microvasculature of the spleen)

     c)   MCHC is elevated in patients with HS. This indicates hyperchromic RBCs, an abnormally high hemoglobin content of the RBC.

      d)   Assess for aplastic crisis (cessation of RBC production).

   4.   Intervention

      a)   Treat acute anemia.

      b)   Promote RBC production and health.

         (1) Give oral folic acid daily to increase RBC production. (Folic acid is required for RBC formation.)

      c)   Prepare for splenectomy to reduce or eliminate hemolysis.

ALERT: In children under 5 years of age, splenectomy is generally avoided because of the increased risk for infection in asplenic children

      d)   Transfusions may be needed if aplastic crisis occurs.

      e)   Provide anticipatory guidance for the patient and family.

         (1) Vaccinations after one has had a splenectomy should include pneumococcal, meningococcal, and *Haemophilus influenzae* type B (Hib) vaccines.

         (2) Review signs and symptoms of acute anemia and when to call health care provider.

         (3) Review importance of prompt notification of health care provider with temperature >101.5 °F in asplenic child (after having had a splenectomy).

  E. β-Thalassemia

    1.   Overview

      a)   Impaired production of the β globin chain of HbA resulting in defective hemoglobin formation. The result is an unstable hemoglobin molecule that is more fragile. RBCs are more fragile; they fail to hold oxygen well, are easily destroyed, and have an unusually shortened lifespan. HbF production increases to compensate.

      b)   Most prevalent among individuals of Mediterranean descent

      c)   Also called thalassemia major or Cooley anemia

    2.   Etiology

      a)   The condition occurs when a child receives a thalassemia gene from each parent.

    3.   Assessment

      a)   As hemolysis increases, the child demonstrates chronic hypoxia and exercise intolerance. Note an abnormal hemoglobin level of 5 to 9 g/dl.

b) Hemosiderosis (excess iron storage in the tissues)/ hemochromatosis (excess iron storage with resultant cellular damage) can occur with increased blood transfusions; iron is a byproduct of the breakdown of RBCs that occurs in RBC hemolysis.

   (1) Observe for bronze skin.

   (2) Assess cardiac status because of iron buildup on heart muscles causing heart failure.

c) As bone marrow attempts to compensate, hyperplasia of the bone marrow cavity may occur, resulting in thinning of the cortex and bone pain; assess for bone pain.

   (1) Assess for skeletal deformities and frontal bossing.

d) Assess for splenomegaly and hepatomegaly.

e) Assess for delayed sexual maturation.

4. Interventions

   a) Administer regular transfusion therapy.

   b) Administer iron chelation therapy, such as Desferal, to remove excess iron.

   c) Be aware of the possibility of pathologic fractures.

   d) Prepare the child and family for a possible splenectomy.

F. Sickle cell disease

1. Overview

   a) Sickle cell disease (SCD) is a term used to describe a group of genetic disorders of hemoglobin production characterized by a predominance of the abnormal hemoglobin S.

   b) SCD, an autosomal recessive hemolytic anemia, is one of the most common genetic diseases in the United States, occurring in 1 in 375 African American live births.

   c) One in 12 African Americans in the United States carries the trait for SCD.

   d) Populations most commonly affected with SCD are those from Africa, the Mediterranean, India, and the Middle East.

2. Pathophysiology

   a) Globin molecule contains the defect in SCD (referred to as HbS); there is an amino acid substitution in the sixth position of the hemoglobin gene.

   b) RBCs containing HbS maintain a relatively normal shape when oxygenated, but change to a sickled shape after giving up oxygen to the tissues of the body.

     c)   RBC sickling is reversible (for a period of time) under conditions of adequate oxygenation and hydration.

     d)   Sickled RBCs are stiff and nonpliable and have difficulty passing through small vessels, resulting in RBC trapping in the narrow vasculature, which impedes blood flow and results in vaso-occlusion, tissue ischemia, and infarction.

     e)   RBC lifespan is reduced from 120 days to 20 days, resulting in anemia.

     f)   Four most common types of SCD (described by their genotypes) are
        (1) SS
        (2) SC
        (3) $S\beta^+$
        (4) $S\beta^0$

     g)   Individuals with sickle cell trait (i.e., carriers for SCD) have one abnormal β globin gene (i.e., S or C) and one normal β globin gene (A).
        (1) Individuals with sickle cell trait experience RBC sickling only under extreme conditions such as extreme dehydration, severe hypoxia, extreme cold or heat.

3. Newborn screening

     a)   Newborn screening for SCD became widespread in the United States in the late 1980s.

     b)   The initial newborn screening is not a confirmatory test. Infants who have abnormal results on newborn screens should have follow-up confirmatory testing and parental screening to distinguish sickle cell trait from SCD.

4. Assessment

     a)   Clinical manifestations of SCD are due to either
        (1) Obstruction by sickled RBCs
        (2) Destruction of RBCs

     b)   Symptoms rarely appear before age 4 months because of the predominance of HbF, which prevents excessive sickling.

     c)   Assess for signs and symptoms of anemia (hemoglobin is typically between 6 and 9 g/dl).

     d)   Assess for pain caused by vaso-occlusive crisis or episode (VOC or VOE) in any site.

e) In infants, assess for dactylitis (hand-foot syndrome), a painful swelling and redness of the hands and feet caused by vaso-occlusion and infarction in the small vessels of the hands and feet. It can be confused with cellulitis, but it is not from an infectious process.

f) Assess for priapism, painful and prolonged erection of the penis caused by vaso-occlusion.

g) Assess for signs of acute chest syndrome. Acute chest syndrome is clinically similar to pneumonia but has more serious complications associated with it, such as marked acute anemia caused by RBC sickling. Pneumococcal pneumonia is common. Assess respiratory status.

h) Assess for signs of infection. Susceptibility to infection begins at about 6 months of age with congestion of the splenic red pulp.

   (1) Fever is the first sign of bacteremia in the child with SCD. A temperature of 101.5 °F or greater requires immediate medical evaluation and treatment because of the risk for overwhelming sepsis.

   (2) Assist in collection of laboratory studies (blood cultures, complete blood cell count, urine, X-ray).

i) Assess for splenic sequestration. Splenic sequestration is a unique problem occurring in patients with SCD causing a trapping of RBCs in the spleen. It occurs most frequently in children 2 months to 5 years with HbSS and may occur into adolescence in children with heterozygous (HbSC) SCD related to the phagocytic filtering properties of the spleen. It can result in hypovolemic shock.

j) Assess for signs of aplastic crisis. Aplastic crisis in the child with SCD is the cessation of RBC production from the bone marrow resulting in profound anemia. Viral infection (particularly human parvovirus) is typically the cause of aplastic crisis in the child with SCD.

k) Assess for delayed growth.

l) Assess for poor wound healing related to decreased peripheral circulation of oxygenated blood.

m) Assess vision related to potential for retinal infarction.

5. Interventions
   a) Pain
      (1) Provide analgesics as ordered.
      (2) Provide nonpharmacologic pain management (e.g., heating pads, massage, distraction).
      (3) Increase hydration (IV + by mouth [PO]) for hemodilution to decrease blood viscosity and reverse VOC.
      (4) Promote oxygenation, especially if pulse oximetry shows oxygen level <95% or 2% below baseline, to decrease ongoing sickling (will not reverse sickled cells).
      (5) Hydroxyurea is a promising new drug being used in research clinical trials to increase the amount of HbF (fetal hemoglobin). The drug is promising in terms of reducing complications of SCD related to VOC and acute chest syndrome.
   b) Acute chest syndrome
      (1) Provide IV antibiotic therapy to treat bacterial infection as a potential source of the acute chest syndrome.
      (2) Promote pulmonary hygiene (chest physiotherapy, cough, deep breathing, mobility)—promotes aeration of the lung and decreases sickling and consequent respiratory distress.
      (3) Administer packed RBCs for severe anemia (<5-6 g/dl)—anemia in acute chest syndrome can be profound.
      (4) Carefully monitor IV fluids—although IV fluids can promote thinning of blood and decreased sickling of RBCs, fluid overload will increase respiratory effort.
      (5) For chest pain, promote splinting of the chest when coughing.
      (6) Promote frequent use of incentive spirometry and mobility to promote lung expansion.
   c) Infection
      (1) Provide IV antibiotics.
         (*a*) Antibiotic IV therapy is required for children with SCD who have a temperature of 101 °F.
         (*b*) Ceftriaxone is often used in children who are at low risk for sepsis while awaiting complete blood cell count and blood culture results.

      d) Splenic sequestration
- (1) Monitor blood pressure to assess for hypovolemia.
- (2) Administer IV fluids and packed RBCs to correct hypovolemia and anemia.
- (3) Consider splenectomy for repeated episodes of splenic sequestration.

      e) Aplastic crisis
- (1) Administer packed RBCs for profound anemia.

      f) Other
- (1) Provide good skin care.
- (2) Avoid aspirin, as it enhances acidosis and promotes sickling.
- (3) Implement relaxation techniques to decrease the child's stress level.
- (4) Try to maintain an HbS level of less than 30% with transfusions to reduce the risk of stroke.
- (5) Initiate genetic counseling.
- (6) Teach the child to avoid activities that promote a crisis, such as excessive exercise, mountain climbing, or deep sea diving; avoid extreme heat or cold.
- (7) Teach the family to seek early treatment of illness to prevent dehydration
- (8) Encourage the child to receive the pneumococcal vaccine.
- (9) Teach child to avoid wearing tight clothing that impedes circulation.

G. Hyperbilirubinemia
1. Overview
      a) Hyperbilirubinemia is a normal occurrence in the newborn.
      b) The liver is not usually mature at birth and produces fewer enzymes.
      c) Decreased enzyme production prevents the breakdown of unconjugated or indirect bilirubin so that it cannot be excreted.
      d) Note: if jaundice appears in the first 24 hours of life or lasts >1 week in a term infant, contact a physician to assess for biliary atresia or hemolytic disease.
2. Assessment
      a) Note jaundice of skin and eyes.

      b) Assess serum indirect bilirubin level, which rises to 12 to 15 mg/dl.

         (1) When blood is drawn, turn off phototherapy lights and transport blood in a covered tube.

      c) Monitor for kernicterus, which occurs when serum indirect bilirubin content is so high that it deposits in the brain cells, resulting in permanent brain damage.

         (1) Assess neurologic status.

      d) Assess hydration status and stooling pattern while infant is in phototherapy.

      e) Assess body temperature when infant is receiving phototherapy.

   3. Interventions

      a) Initiate phototherapy; use bilirubin reduction lights to decompose unconjugated bilirubin beneath the skin, promoting excretion.

      b) During phototherapy reposition frequently.

      c) Maintain normal body temperature and adequate hydration.

      d) If using conventional bilirubin lights

         (1) Keep the lights at least 12 in. away from the infant.

         (2) Keep the child's eyes shielded from the light at all times.

         (3) Keep the child naked.

         (4) Infant may be removed for a maximum of 20 minutes per feeding.

      e) If using a fiberoptic blanket, keep the infant wrapped in it at all times, including during feeding; eye patches are not necessary but may be used if the family is concerned.

         (1) A phototherapy-compatible diaper may be used for monitoring output.

      f) Assist with an exchange transfusion if the child does not respond to phototherapy.

IV. Disease conditions affecting the clotting cascade

  A. Altered clotting function

    1. Platelets (thrombocytes) overview

      a) Platelets are the smallest of the formed elements in the blood.

         (1) They are not nucleated.

         (2) They live 4 to 10 days.

(3) Normal platelet values in children are between 150,000 and 400,000/mm³.

b) Platelets cause capillary homeostasis by adhering to the inner surface of a vessel and sticking to each other.

(1) They produce a temporary mechanical plug.

(2) They repair breaks in small blood vessels and capillaries, especially in the skin, mucous membranes, and internal organs.

c) Heparin, aspirin, guaifenesin (Robitussin), indomethacin (Indocin), and phenylbutazone (Butazolidin) interfere with platelet function.

2. Normal clotting mechanism

a) In the intrinsic pathway, platelet factor, antihemophilic (factor VIII), and multiple clotting factors (including calcium) result in thromboplastin formation; generation of thromboplastin is measured by partial thromboplastin time (PTT).

b) In the extrinsic pathway, injured cells release incomplete thromboplastin; this plus multiple clotting factors results in thromboplastin formation.

c) Prothrombin and vitamin K (with the help of thromboplastin) result in thrombin production, which is measured by prothrombin time (PT).

d) Fibrinogen, thrombin, and factor VIII result in a fibrin clot, which is measured by thrombin time.

B. Idiopathic thrombocytopenic purpura

1. Overview

a) Idiopathic thrombocytopenic purpura (ITP) is an acquired hemorrhagic disorder that results in the autoimmune destruction of platelets in the spleen.

b) ITP is typically proceeded by an upper respiratory tract infection or other viral illness.

2. Assessment

a) Clinical manifestations are consistent with those found in profound thrombocytopenia because the platelet count in ITP is typically <20,000/mm³.

(1) Assess for petechial rash.

(2) Note bruises and other signs of bleeding such as blood in the urine or from gums.

3. Interventions

a) Provide oral steroid therapy for platelet count >20,000/mm³ to stop the autoimmune assault on platelets.

b) Administer IV immunoglobulins for platelet count <20,000/mm³.

c) Administer platelet transfusions, if ordered.

d) Consider splenectomy for prolonged ITP unresponsive to treatment.

e) Provide for safety measures to prevent trauma and bleeding, such as avoiding contact sports.

f) Avoid using injections; if one is necessary, inject subcutaneously and hold pressure for 5 minutes.

g) Do not administer aspirin, which increases bleeding.

C. Hemophilia
1. Overview
   a) Hemophilia comprises a group of disorders that result from a deficiency in one of the clotting factors; it is not a platelet deficiency.

   b) The most common type (75% of all cases) is hemophilia A (also called factor VIII deficiency or classic hemophilia), a sex-linked recessive disorder.

   c) Other common types are hemophilia B (also called factor IX deficiency or Christmas disease) and hemophilia C (factor XI deficiency).

   d) Hemophilia is classified according to the presence of factor activity. Each severity level is a predictor of the ease with which a child is prone to bleeding.

Severity	Factor activity	Bleeding tendency
Severe	1%	Spontaneous bleeding without trauma
Moderate	1%-5%	Bleeding with trauma
Mild	5%-50%	Bleeding with severe trauma or surgery

2. Genetics
   a) Genetic counseling should be offered to affected parents.
   (1) If the father has the disorder and the mother does not, all daughters will be carriers, but sons will not have the disease.
   (2) If the mother is a carrier and the father does not have hemophilia, each son has a 50% chance of getting hemophilia and each daughter has a 50% chance of being a carrier.

3. Assessment
   a) Assess for signs of bleeding, especially after circumcision, immunizations, or minor injuries.
      (1) Multiple bruises without petechiae
      (2) Multiple episodes of hemarthrosis (joint bleeding)
         (a) Measure the joint's circumference and compare with that of the unaffected joint.
         (b) Note swelling, pain, or impaired joint mobility.
         (c) Assess for joint degeneration from repeated hemarthrosis.
      (3) Assess for bleeding into the neck, mouth, and thorax, which can seriously threaten respiratory status.
      (4) Check for peripheral neuropathies from bleeding near peripheral nerves.
   b) Assess for decreased clotting factor levels and prolonged PTT.
   c) Assess HIV status, as there is a very small increased risk of HIV in recipients of clotting factor.
4. Interventions
   a) Interventions to prevent bleeding
      (1) Consider helmet use in toddler with moderate to severe hemophilia.
      (2) Pad toys and other objects in child's environment.
      (3) Recommend Toothettes (instead of bristle toothbrushes) and stool softeners if needed.
      (4) Encourage activities that do not involve contact or the potential for injury, such as chess, fishing, theater. (Avoid contact sports.)
      (5) Discourage weight gain and obesity, which would increase the load of the joints.
      (6) Give IV factor replacement to maintain an acceptable serum level of cryoprecipitate or frozen factor VIII; this is usually done by the family at home.
   b) Interventions when bleeding occurs
      (1) Instruct the family to give factor replacement as soon as possible to minimize bleeding.
      (2) Elevate the affected extremity above the heart.
      (3) Immobilize the site to facilitate the clot forming.

(4) Avoid aspirin or other medications or treatments (sutures, cauterization) that may intensify or aggravate the bleeding.

(5) Perform bilateral site assessments and circumference measurements when there is an unaffected site for comparison.

c) Interventions for hemarthrosis

(1) Immobilize the affected extremity.

(2) Promote vasoconstriction by applying ice compresses and pressure and by administering hemostatic agents, such as fibrin foam or topical adrenaline or epinephrine.

(3) Treat pain as needed.

(4) Avoid excessive movement or weight bearing for 48 hours.

(5) Begin mild range-of-motion exercises after 48 hours to facilitate absorption and prevent contractures.

(6) Decrease anxiety to lower the child's heart rate.

CHAPTER

6

Infectious Diseases

LEARNING OBJECTIVES

1. Describe the five methods of obtaining immune protection against communicable diseases.

2. Discuss vaccine types and their major side effects.

3. List the suggested immunization schedule and its rationale.

4. Identify the most common communicable childhood diseases that immunization can prevent.

I. Chapter overview

Infectious diseases are common among children. A child receives protection from communicable diseases naturally or artificially. Immunizations of various types are given at specific times to protect the child from certain diseases.

II. Methods of obtaining immune protection

A. Natural (innate)
   1. This protection, present at birth, is not learned and does not depend on prior contact.
   2. Examples of natural immunity include barriers against disease, such as skin and mucous membranes, and bacteriocidal substances of body fluids, such as intestinal flora and gastric acidity.
   3. Some species are naturally immune to some diseases.

B. Naturally acquired active
   1. The immune system actively makes antibodies after exposure to disease.
   2. This protection lasts for life.
   3. A high risk of side effects exists, because the child contracts the disease.

C. Naturally acquired passive
   1. No active immune process is involved; the antibodies are passively received.
   2. The antibodies are acquired through placental transfer via IgG (the smallest immunoglobulin) and breast-feeding (colostrum).

D. Artificially acquired active
   1. Medically engineered substances are inhaled or injected to stimulate the immune response against a specific disease.
   2. Examples include all immunizations.

E. Artificially acquired passive
   1. Antibodies are injected without stimulating the immune response.
   2. The antibodies are used as antitoxins or for prophylaxis.
   3. The antibodies provide immediate protection that lasts for weeks.
   4. Examples include gamma globulin (a mixture of antibodies against disease that are prevalent in the community, pooled from 8,000 donors of human plasma) and hyperimmune

or convalescent serum globulin (such as tetanus immune globulin, hepatitis B immune globulin, and varicella-zoster immune globulin).

III. Stages of infectious diseases

A. Incubation period: the time between the invasion of the organism and the development of infection with the organism; a time of replication of the organism within the body

B. Prodromal period: the time between the onset of nonspecific signs and symptoms such as fever and malaise and the disease-specific symptoms

C. Communicability period: the stage when the disease is transmissible to others (i.e., contagious)

D. Illness stage: the period when disease-specific symptoms are manifested

E. Convalescent period: the time between the disappearance of disease-specific symptoms and the complete return to wellness

IV. Types of vaccines

A. Live, attenuated
  1. A live organism, grown under suboptimal conditions, results in a live vaccine with reduced virulence.
  2. The vaccine confers 90% to 95% protection for 20+ years with a single dose, although some now need a booster.
  3. It promotes a full range of immunologic responses.
  4. The organisms for the vaccine are modified by heat or chemicals but still retain their ability to replicate and stimulate immunity.
  5. Examples include measles, mumps, and rubella (MMR) vaccine, varicella vaccine, and the nasal influenza vaccine spray.

B. Inactivated
  1. An inactivated vaccine offers a weaker response than a live vaccine, necessitating frequent boosters.
  2. A toxoid is treated with formalin or heat and rendered nontoxic but still antigenic; it provides 90% to 100% protection.
  3. A killed vaccine does not promote replication because it only involves the cell wall; it provides 40% to 70% protection.

4. Genetically engineered/recombinant DNA technology can use the smallest part of the antigen needed to stimulate immunity, thus significantly decreasing the side effects.
   a) The diffusible fraction of a virus is the part of the microorganism capable of inducing immunity.
5. Examples of inactivated vaccines include the diphtheria and tetanus toxoids, the acellular pertussis vaccine, inactivated polio vaccine, hepatitis B vaccine, and the influenza vaccine.

V. Vaccines

A. Schedule
   1. See Table 1, Child and Adolescent Immunizations 2006 Fact Sheet. Yearly updates can be viewed at www.cdc.gov/nip

B. Timing of doses and cautions
   1. Vaccines generally require at least 4 weeks between doses; some require more.
   2. Boosters are used to maintain optimal titers of antibodies by stimulating antigenic memory.
      a) The primary response takes 10 to14 days to develop an antibody titer.
      b) The booster response takes 1 to 3 days to reach a high antibody titer.
      c) Boosters are determined to provide the optimal protection during a time when the child is at the greatest risk for suffering the sequelae of the disease.
   3. Review the child's immunization status at every health encounter.
   4. Recognize a child's need for immunization on the basis of knowledge of the most current child and adolescent immunization schedule by the Centers for Disease Control and Prevention (CDC).
   5. If the schedule is interrupted, do not repeat earlier doses; continue the schedule according to previous guidelines.
   6. Identify contraindications to the administration of given vaccines and seek further evaluation of the child before immunizations are given. These include the following:
      a) A history of life-threatening reaction or allergy to a previous dose of the vaccine; ask which side effects (if any) the child had from the last immunization and when the symptoms occurred.

        b)   Moderate to severe acute illness; do not vaccinate if the child has an elevated temperature; this side effect of the vaccine would be difficult to differentiate from an exacerbation of the original condition.

           (1) Reschedule vaccine administration when the child is well.

        c)   Immune suppression (including receipt of chemotherapy or gamma globulin within the past 6 weeks).

        d)   Pregnancy

7.   Administer the greatest possible number of immunizations at each health encounter; all active vaccines may be administered simultaneously with different needles and at different sites.

        a)   Use vastus lateralis (anterior aspect of the thigh) site in the infant and young child for most vaccines; avoid dorsogluteal and deltoid sites in infants because of small muscle mass and the potential for nerve damage.

        b)   Multiple vaccine administration is safe and does not increase the likelihood of experiencing side effects.

8.   Side effects from bacterial vaccines typically occur within hours and days of the vaccine; side effects from live virus vaccines typically occur 2 to 4 weeks after administration.

9.   Withhold the pertussis vaccine if the child has a progressive and active central nervous system problem; the child with cerebral palsy can receive all vaccines.

10. The first MMR vaccination is scheduled between 12 and 15 months to prevent interference with maternal antibodies that develop a protective titer.

        a)   During an epidemic, give the measles vaccine to the child as young as age 6 months, but this dose will not count toward the two required doses.

11. Active and passive vaccines are seldom given at the same time, except for tetanus, because a passive vaccine can inhibit the production of a protective titer.

12. Cutting doses in half is not effective and does not count as a dose of the immunization (two halves do not equal one whole dose); dividing doses does not decrease the incidence of side effects.

13. Do not give the tuberculosis (TB) purified protein derivative test and the measles vaccine at the same time; the measles vaccine may make a TB-positive individual appear to be TB negative.

14. Illness with Hib in the young child does not confer immunity; immunization is still required through age 5.
15. Vaccines are no longer given when the risk of side effects is greater than the risk of sequelae from getting the disease.
16. Pediatric vaccines no longer contain thimerosal because of mercury and its potential effect on neurologic development.

C. Storage of vaccines
1. Ensure potency of vaccines by checking expiration dates and storing vaccines in the middle shelf of the refrigerator, not on the door.
2. Light can inactivate the MMR vaccine viruses. Once reconstituted, protect from light, refrigerate but do not freeze, and use within 8 hours.
3. Influenza vaccine should never be frozen.
4. Varicella vaccine should be frozen and protected from light; it can be refrigerated for 72 hours; once reconstituted, use within 30 minutes.

D. Parent-child education
1. Review Vaccine Information Sheets provided by the CDC; these include purpose and side effects (see Table 1).
2. Review administration of antipyretics such as acetaminophen and other comfort measures related to potential vaccine side effects.
3. Review when to call the health care provider:
   a) Signs and symptoms of severe adverse reaction
      (1) Difficulty breathing
      (2) Hoarseness or wheezing
      (3) Hives
      (4) Pallor
      (5) Lethargy
      (6) Dizziness
      (7) Tachycardia
   b) High fever
   c) Behavioral changes
   d) Any concerns
4. On the basis of the immunization schedule, inform parents of what immunizations are next and when they should be administered.
5. For children born abroad, vaccines and routes of administration may vary widely with those acceptable in the United States. Parents may question the number, frequency, and route of vaccinations required in the United States.

VI. Bacterial infections

A. Diphtheria
   1. Caused by bacteria that proliferate in the respiratory tract and multiply on dead tissue in the throat, producing exotoxin and exudate consisting of a tough fibrous membrane (pseudomembrane) across the respiratory tract; this results in mechanical airway obstruction
   2. More serious in infants
   3. Can cause renal, cardiac, and peripheral central nervous system damage
   4. Rare; 0 to 2 cases in the United States each year

B. Tetanus (lockjaw)
   1. It is caused by anaerobic spore-forming bacteria that produce an exotoxin, which is present in soil, house dust, and animal feces.
   2. The exotoxin is introduced through the skin.
   3. It reaches the axons of the nerves, causing voluntary muscle contraction, muscular rigidity, and painful paroxysmal seizures.
   4. There is no transplacental immunity; attacks are equally dangerous to adults and children.
   5. There are <40 cases of tetanus a year in the United States, but the mortality rate is 18%.
   6. First symptoms are trismus (lockjaw) and difficulty swallowing.
   7. It can cause laryngospasm, respiratory distress, intramuscular hemorrhage, and death.
   8. Interventions are as follows:
      a) If the child has a clean wound, has completed the primary series, and has boosters less than 10 years old, no treatment is needed other than cleaning the wound.
      b) If the wound is contaminated, the immunization series is complete, and immunization was >5 years ago, administer a toxoid (Td).
      c) If the child has a contaminated wound and an incomplete initial series of immunizations, or if the child's immunizations are more than 10 years old, give the toxoid and immunoglobulin.

C. Pertussis (whooping cough)
   1. Pertussis is caused by bacteria that proliferate in the respiratory tract.

2. It is transmitted primarily by intimate respiratory contact and is highly contagious.

3. There were 19,000 cases in 2004 in the United States.

4. The classic sign is paroxysmal or spasmodic cough that ends in a prolonged inspiratory whoop; cough can last for weeks.

5. Respiratory distress can result in anoxia during coughing spasms, with cyanosis and loss of consciousness.

6. The disease can result in encephalopathy (seizures, apnea, mental retardation, hernia, stroke), pneumonia, and death (risk of death decreases with increasing age).

7. Interventions are as follows:

   a) Maintain patent airway; keep suctioning and ventilation (bag and mask) equipment available.

   b) Maintain bed rest until coughing subsides.

   c) Anticipate use of a mist tent to loosen secretions.

   d) Administer erythromycin as ordered.

D. Hib

   1. Prior to the vaccine, Hib was the leading cause of serious bacterial disease (bacterial meningitis, epiglottitis, sepsis, and cellulitis) in U.S. children under 5 years of age.

      a) Sixty percent of those affected are under 1 year of age.

      b) Hib is not common in older children and adults; most Hib disease strikes infants who are not immunized; especially common in day care settings.

      c) Transmission is through respiratory droplets; rarely spread through contact with environmental surface.

   2. Mortality rate is 3% to 7% with increased morbidity (deafness, mental retardation, ataxia).

E. Sepsis (septicemia)

   1. General information

      a) The condition involves a generalized bacterial infection in the bloodstream.

      b) Infants, particularly under 1 month of age, are at risk because of their immature immune systems.

      c) Mortality related to sepsis has diminished, but the incidence remains constant.

      d) Group B streptococci and *Escherichia coli* are the most common causes of neonatal sepsis.

   2. Assessment

      a) Neonates and young infants

(1) Prodromal stage
   (*a*) Fever or hypothermia
   (*b*) Poor feeding
   (*c*) Lethargy/increased sleeping
   (*d*) Irritability
(2) Illness stage
   (*a*) Pallor
   (*b*) Cyanosis
   (*c*) Temperature instability
   (*d*) Tachycardia
   (*e*) Hypotension
   (*f*) Apnea
   (*g*) Dehydration
   (*h*) Tense fontanel
   (*i*) Seizures

b) Children
  (1) Prodromal stage
    (*a*) Fever
    (*b*) Malaise
    (*c*) Stiff neck
    (*d*) Headache

3. Interventions
  a) Monitor and support cardiorespiratory function.
    (1) Provide airway/ventilation equipment at the bedside.
    (2) Monitor for signs and symptoms of shock such as decreased level of consciousness and hypotension; note that hypotension is a late and ominous sign in the pediatric patient.
  b) Assist with collection of blood, urine, and cerebrospinal fluid cultures as needed.
  c) Administer antibiotic therapy as ordered.

F. Tuberculosis
  1. Overview
    a) TB is caused by *Mycobacterium tuberculosis.*
    b) It is transferred by respiratory spread, usually from a household member or someone frequently in the home or school.
    c) It can be in the lungs or disseminate to other sites, such as the brain, bone, and kidneys; dissemination is called miliary TB.

    d) High-risk groups that should be tested include those with known contact with someone with TB, children who were born in or have traveled to countries where TB is endemic, and those exposed to adults engaging in high-risk activities (IV drug use) or in high-risk environments (jails, homeless settings, migrant farm workers).

  2. Assessment

    a) Most children are asymptomatic.

    b) Symptoms may reflect the organ involved or may appear as flu symptoms.

  3. First indication may be a positive purified protein derivative tuberculin test/Mantoux test (PPD).

 Note: The 4-prong tine test is no longer used in the United States.

    a) A positive reaction is indicated by the area of induration (raised area) and *not* the area of redness.

    b) A positive reaction can *only* be read from 48 to 72 hours after the intradermal skin test is administered; earlier swelling is a neutrophil response and is not related to tuberculin antibodies.

    c) A positive reaction does not indicate that a person has active disease; it only indicates that he or she has been exposed.

    d) After a positive PPD, further testing by X-ray and for the presence of the organism in culture is needed.

  4. Interventions

    a) First-line drugs include isoniazid, rifampin, and streptomycin.

    b) These cases are reported to the public health department; it will provide guidance if any environmental restrictions are needed.

VII. Viral infections

 A. Rubeola (measles)

  1. Respiratory tract virus that lasts 10 days; highly contagious

  2. Prodromal symptoms: fever; malaise; a harsh, rasping cough; conjunctivitis; and coryza

  3. Later symptoms: maculopapular, red, pruritic rash; photophobia; and Koplik's spots on the buccal mucosa

4. Potential consequences: bacterial superinfections, such as pneumonia and encephalitis with possible retardation, subacute sclerosing panencephalitis, and death

B. Rubella (German measles)
1. Respiratory tract virus that lasts 3 days
2. Symptoms: subauricular and suboccipital lymphadenopathy; a pink, mild maculopapular rash
3. Potential consequences: arthralgia and arthritis, idiopathic thrombocytopenia purpura, and encephalitis.
4. Congenital rubella syndrome
   a) Seen in infants whose mothers contracted rubella during pregnancy.
   b) Results in growth retardation, mental retardation, cataracts, deafness, and cardiac anomalies

C. Parotitis (mumps)
1. Respiratory tract virus, usually lasting 7 to 10 days
2. Symptoms: swelling in the parotid glands and painful swallowing
3. Potential consequences: aseptic meningitis, orchitis, and epididymitis in older males, nerve deafness, and encephalitis

D. Poliomyelitis (polio)
1. Fecal-oral enterovirus that replicates in the gastrointestinal tract and then enters the blood; spread by contaminated saliva, feces, sewage, or water
2. Symptoms: initially, a stiff neck and muscle pains, followed by nerve cell damage and asymmetrical flaccid paralysis; no sensory deficit
3. No recent cases of polio in the United States but still common in other countries
4. Oral, live attenuated vaccine no longer given in United States because of live virus being excreted in stool and resulting in vaccine-associated paralytic polio in unprotected individuals

E. Varicella (chickenpox)
1. Respiratory herpes zoster virus; no protection provided from maternal antibodies.
2. Highly contagious from 1 to 2 days before the appearance of a rash until all the blisters are all dried up, which usually takes 4 to 6 days after the rash appears; incubation period = 21 days

3. Symptoms: pruritic vesicular rash beginning on the trunk and going proximodistally
    a) The lesions occur in all stages at the same time; they then crust and scab.
    b) The scabs are not infectious.
    c) The child may return to school when all of the lesions have scabbed.
4. Potential consequences: bacterial superinfections, pneumonia, encephalitis, Reye syndrome, and shingles
5. Interventions: keep the child's nails short, pat (do not rub) the sores, apply calamine lotion, give lukewarm oatmeal baths, administer antihistamines, and dress the child in light, loose-fitting clothes
6. Do not give aspirin or other salicylates. There is a high association between the administration of aspirin during varicella infection and the development of Reye syndrome, an acute encephalopathy with cerebral cortex swelling but without inflammation, accompanied by fatty changes in the liver and impaired liver function and hyperammonemia.

F. Fifth disease (erythema infectiosum)
1. Caused by parvovirus B19
2. Transmission by droplet
3. Incubation of 6 to 14 days
4. Signs and symptoms: intensely red facial rash, forming a "slapped face" appearance that eventually fades; rash on the extensor surfaces of extremities 1 day later and lasting 1 or more weeks
5. Interventions: comfort measures, analgesics as ordered, cutting child's fingernails to avoid injury from scratching, lukewarm water baths with baking soda or oatmeal to soothe itching

G. Mononucleosis
1. A self-limiting viral infection spread among monocytes; transmitted by direct contact of oropharyngeal secretions
2. Can be caused by the Epstein-Barr virus
3. Incubation period of 2 to 6 weeks
4. Prevalent among adolescents, but can occur in young children
5. Signs and symptoms: complete blood cell count shows atypical monocytes, positive Monospot test, splenomegaly, hepatomegaly, possible lymph node enlargement, sore throat, and lethargy

6. Interventions: comfort measures, rest, fluid intake, avoid contact sports to prevent splenic rupture

H. Neonatal hepatitis B (HBV)
   1. Infants born to HBV-positive mothers have a 70% to 90% risk of HBV infection.
   2. Eighty percent to 90% of infected infants become chronic HBV carriers; more than 25% of these infants die of primary hepatocellular carcinoma or cirrhosis.

I. Roseola infantum
   1. Caused by herpesvirus 6
   2. Incubation of approximately 10 days
   3. Unknown mode of transmission
   4. Signs and symptoms: high fever, irritability, and discrete rose-pink macule appearing after abrupt fall in fever, most often on trunk and fading under pressure
   5. Interventions: antipyretics as ordered for fever, cool compresses and sponge baths to reduce fever, comfort measures

VIII. Pneumococcal disease

A. This is now the most common cause of vaccine-preventable death.

B. It causes meningitis, sepsis, pneumococcal pneumonia, ear infections.

C. There is increased incidence in day care settings.

D. There is increased incidence of antibiotic resistance.

E. Pneumococcus is also known as streptococcal pneumonia.

F. There are 90 different serotypes, but 7 account for 80% of invasive disease.

G. The disease is spread by respiratory droplets.

IX. Tick-carried infection

A. Lyme disease
   1. The most common tick-borne disorder
   2. Symptoms
      a) Tick bite followed in 3 to 32 days by erythema at the bite site; this area increases in size to look like a doughnut with raised edges; rash may be warm and pruritic.
      b) Development of headache, fatigue, anorexia, stiff neck, and fever

      c)   Progresses to systemic involvement 2 to 11 weeks later
- (1) Neurologic symptoms (Bell's palsy, aseptic meningitis)
- (2) Cardiac conduction problems
- (3) Musculoskeletal symptoms (arthritis)

  3.   Interventions
      a)   Prevention is the best treatment.
- (1) Wear long pants and shirt while in wooded areas.
- (2) Shower with soap after being in wooded areas or near outside pets that have been in these areas.

      b)   Administer antibiotics (amoxicillin or erythromycin)

B. Rocky Mountain Spotted Fever

  1.   The most common rickettsial disease in the United States

  2.   Transmitted by tick most often in the spring and early summer

  3.   Can be fatal if left untreated

  4.   Symptoms
      a)   History of a tick bite
      b)   Severe headache
      c)   Measleslike rash beginning as bright red macules on ankles and wrists, spreading as a hemorrhagic rash to the palms, soles, back, arms, thighs, and chest

  5.   Interventions
      a)   Removal of tick slowly and steadily
      b)   Cleansing wound with soap and water
      c)   Administering tetracycline as ordered

Table 1. Child and adolescent immunizations 2006/fact sheet

Vaccine	Schedule	Specific contraindications	Common side effects	Severe adverse reactions	Important facts
Hepatitis A (Hep A)	Dose 1: 12-23 months Dose 2: at least 6 months later	None	Soreness at administration site Headache Loss of appetite Tiredness	Rare	Not licensed for children under 1 year Safety of administration during pregnancy unknown
Hepatitis B (Hep B)	Dose 1: birth Dose 2: 1-2 months Dose 3: 6-18 months	Previous history of a life-threatening allergic reaction to baker's yeast (as in bread)	Soreness at administration site Mild to moderate fever	Very rare	Individuals > 18 years of age in high-risk groups should also receive this vaccine
Haemophilus influenzae, type B (Hib)	Dose 1: 2 months Dose 2: 4 months Dose 3: 6 months Dose 4: 12-15 months.	<6 weeks of age	Redness, warmth, swelling at the site Fever >101°F, may last 2-3 days	None	Protects against bacterial meningitis, epiglottitis, bacterial pneumonia, septic arthritis, and sepsis Conjugated vaccine
Polio (IPV) (inactivated polio vaccine)	Dose 1: 2 months Dose 2: 4 months Dose 3: 6-18 months Dose 4: 4-6 years	Previous history of a life-threatening allergic reaction to the antibiotics: neomycin, streptomycin, and polymyxin B	Soreness at site (uncommon)	None	IPV is used exclusively in the United States because of a small incidence of vaccine-associated polio paralysis (VAPP) associated with the live oral vaccine.
Diphtheria, tetanus, and acellular pertussis (DTaP)	Dose 1: 2 months Dose 2: 4 months Dose 3: 6 months Dose 4: 15-18 months Dose 5: 4-6 years NEW: Tdap at age 11-12 if they have not received the Td (below)	Previous history of brain or nervous system disease within 72 hours after a dose of DTaP	Fever Redness or swelling at the site or of the extremity Soreness at the site	Occur in <1/1 million doses Severe problems that have been reported: • Seizures, coma, or decreased consciousness • Permanent brain damage	Children who have experienced the following after a dose of DTaP should talk with health care provider: • Seizure or collapse • Cried nonstop >3 hours • Temperature >104° F Tdap contains a lowered adult dose of diphtheria and pertussis
Tetanus/ diphtheria Td (adult)	14 to 16 years Repeat every 10 years throughout life		Soreness, redness or swelling at administration site	Very rare Deep aching, pain, and muscle wasting at injection site	Needed throughout life Td contains a lowered adult dose of diphtheria
Tdap (adolescent)	11-12 years	None			Tdap contains a lowered dose of pertussis and diphtheria
Pneumococcal	Dose 1: 2 months Dose 2: 4 months Dose 3: 12-15 months	Hypersensitivity to DTaP and latex	Redness or tenderness at the site (1/4 infants) Low-grade fever (common) High fever (less common) Fussiness, drowsiness, decreased appetite	None	7-valent vaccine given to children; 23-valent vaccine given to adults Especially important for those with chronic conditions, especially asplenia, sickle cell disease, and immune suppression

Measles, mumps, and rubella (MMR)	Dose 1: 12-15 months Dose 2: 4-6 years	Previous history of a life-threatening allergic reaction to gelatin or neomycin. Pregnant women should avoid getting the MMR until after giving birth. Individuals with known conditions (cancer, HIV/AIDS) or who are taking medication that affects the immune system (steroid use for >2 weeks) should check with their health care provider before getting the MMR vaccines.	Fever Mild rash Swelling of cheek or neck glands (rare) Signs and symptoms usually occur within 2 weeks of the MMR. Moderate side effects: • Febrile seizure • Joint pain/stiffness • Temporary low platelet count (thrombocytopenia) • Temporary swelling of the lymph nodes (lymphadenopathy)	Deafness Seizures, coma, or lowered consciousness Encephalitis Permanent brain damage Data are inconclusive and experts disagree about whether or not the vaccine is the causative agent for these reactions.	Women should not get pregnant for 1 month after getting the vaccine. This is a live, attenuated vaccine. MMR does not cause autism, nor does it exacerbate TB. In an outbreak, immunize those <6 months within 72 hours of exposure, but do not count toward the required immunization.
Meningococcal (MCV4)	One dose at 11-12 years or any age up to 55 years	History of Guillain-Barré syndrome (GBS) Allergy to vaccine components	Redness Allergic reaction Fever		Not effective in infants <2 years Especially important for college freshmen Does not last a long time in the system
Varicella	First dose: 12-15 months Second dose: 4-6 years. People over 13 who have not had the vaccine should get 2 doses given 4-8 weeks apart.	Previous history of a life-threatening allergic reaction to gelatin or neomycin. Pregnant women should avoid getting the MMR until after giving birth. Individuals with known conditions (cancer, HIV/AIDS) or who are taking medication that affects the immune system (steroid use for >2 weeks) should check with their health care provider before getting the varicella vaccine.	Soreness or swelling at the site (1/5) Fever (1/10) Mild rash, up to 1 month after the vaccine (<1/20) It is possible for people who have the vaccine-induced rash to infect other household contacts, but it is rare. Moderate side effects: • Febrile seizures (1/1,000)	Pneumonia (rare) Severe brain reactions (extremely rare) Anemia (extremely rare) Data are inconclusive, and experts disagree about whether or not the vaccine is the causative agent for these reactions.	Women should not get pregnant for 1 month after getting the vaccine. Not given before the first birthday
Influenza	First time: 2 doses • Trivalent Inactivated Influenza Vaccine (TIV) ≥4 weeks apart • Live Attenuated Intranasal Vaccine (LAIV) ≥6 weeks apart Annually:1 dose • 6-23 months (healthy) • ≥6 months (at risk; asthma, cardiac disease, sickle cell disease, HIV, diabetes)	TIV • Previous history of life-threatening reaction to eggs or to previous vaccine dose. • History of GBS LAIV • Age <5 years or >49 years • Immune deficiency • Chronic illness • Pregnant women • <18 years of age on long-term aspirin	TIV • Soreness or swelling at the site • Fever • Aches LAIV • Runny nose, nasal congestion, cough • Fever • Headache • Abdominal pain, vomiting, or diarrhea	TIV • GBS (1-2 cases per million) LAIV • None	It is recommended that health care workers receive the TIV. The vaccine is updated yearly to best reflect the strains of influenza that are most prevalent. Only effective for a few months

Because of the annual changes made to the immunization schedule, it is necessary that updated information be obtained from the CDC site at www.cdc.gov/nip.

CHAPTER
7

Immune System Dysfunction

LEARNING OBJECTIVES

1. Discuss conditions associated with alterations in white blood cell function.

2. Plan appropriate nursing interventions for the child with immune suppression.

3. Relate allergy and autoimmune disease to abnormal immune function.

4. Discuss different types of allergy.

I. Chapter overview

Knowledge of normal white blood cell and immune function provides the foundation for understanding the conditions associated with altered immunologic function. Assessment and intervention are geared to controlling the problems associated with the alteration and promoting normal function. Prevention plays a primary role in hypersensitivity reactions.

II. Alterations in white blood cell (WBC) formation and immune functioning

A. Immune system components
1. Primary lymphoid organs include the thymus, bone marrow, and liver.
2. Secondary lymphoid organs include the spleen, lymph nodes, and gut-associated lymphoid tissues.

B. Human leukocyte antigen (HLA)
1. Is a major histocompatibility complex normally found on the cell surface of every nucleated cell (not on RBCs)
2. Allows the body to recognize self versus nonself; consists of four main loci (HLA-A, HLA-B, HLA-C, HLA-D/DR)
   a) For organ transplants, markers are matched as closely as possible to decrease the odds of rejection.
   b) The cornea is avascular and thus does not require HLA matching.
3. Is genetically passed on chromosome 6, so the child gets markers from both parents
4. Contains a genetic predisposition or susceptibility to a disorder; does not pass the disorder itself
5. There is a 1-in-30,000 chance that two nonrelated people have the same HLA

C. Immune system function
1. Defense against nonself antigens
   a) Hyperfunctioning results in allergy.
   b) Hypofunctioning results in an immunodeficiency.
2. Homeostasis
   a) Homeostasis involves the phagocytosis of debris from cellular warfare or of dead cells; this is nature's way to clean out dead debris from the system.
   b) Hyperfunction results in autoimmune disease.
3. Surveillance against any antigenic invasion; hypofunctioning results in cancer

D. Natural first line of defense against infection
1. Skin
2. Body secretions (tears, saliva, sebum, mucus, acidic environments, normal body flora, and salt in sweat)
3. Nasal hairs and cilia
4. Controlled body temperature
5. Adequate renal function

E. Immune cells and their function
1. Neutrophil (polymorphonuclear leukocyte): a short-lived phagocyte that is the first immune cell at the site of inflammation, infection, or trauma
   a) It attacks bacteria and fungi.
   b) A band is an immature cell; a segmented neutrophil (seg) is a mature cell.
   c) Neutrophils make up 60% of the WBC count.
2. Eosinophil: effective in phagocytizing parasites; also stimulates inflammation, especially in response to mast cell degranulation, and increases with allergic attack (1%-3% of WBCs)
3. Basophil: releases histamine, heparin, and other substances during an allergic attack (<0.1% of WBCs)
   a) It is responsible for many symptoms of anaphylaxis.
   b) In the tissues, it is known as mast cells; especially prevalent in the eyes, ears, nose, and throat and under the skin.
4. Monocyte: phagocytizes antigens and presents antigenic markers to lymphocytes so that antibodies can be made (3%-7% of WBCs)
   a) It appears later than a neutrophil but lasts longer.
   b) It includes Kupffer cells of the liver.
   c) A macrophage is a monocyte that has left the circulation and entered the tissues.
   d) It releases cytokines to attract other immune cells to the site of attack.
   e) An increase indicates chronic inflammation.
5. B lymphocyte
   a) IgM is the largest immunoglobulin (Ig); it stays in the blood, activates complement, and is responsible for making antibodies against the ABO blood groups.
   b) IgG is the smallest Ig and the only one that passes through the placenta, thus offering the newborn passive protection; it activates complement and has an excellent memory.

  c) IgD is a lymphocyte receptor whose action is not well understood.

  d) Secretory IgA is present in all body secretions; including breast milk, saliva, and tears; it prevents viruses from entering through the mucous membranes.

  e) IgE governs the allergic response by stimulating basophils to release their products after contact with the allergen.

 6. T lymphocyte (T cell): carries out functions directly or by its cells' products; releases soluble factors (lymphokines) that stimulate the immune system; all T cells are processed through the thymus.

  a) CD4 cells (helper T cells, Th) tell the B cells when to make antibodies and how many to make.

  b) CD8 cells (suppressor T, Ts, or cytotoxic T cells) tell the B cells to stop making antibodies.

  c) Normally there are twice as many CD4 as CD8 cells, so the system is always in a state of readiness.

  d) There are two subsets of CD4: Th1 and Th2.

   (1) Increased Th2 has an increased role in the allergic response.

   (2) Those with high Th1 do not have allergy.

 7. Lymphocytes make up 25% to 33% of the WBCs.

 8. The normal WBC count = 4.5 to 13.5×10^3 cells/mm^3.

 9. Function of immune cells in the inflammatory reaction is as follows:

  a) Histamine causes vasodilation, and granulocytes and monocytes are attracted to the site.

  b) Cells leave the blood and enter the damaged site, resulting in redness, warmth, swelling, pain, and altered function.

III. Fever

 A. Introduction

  1. Fever is a normal body response to assist the immune system in destroying foreign antigens.

  2. Temperatures of less than 100.4-101 °F (38-38.5 °C) usually do not require treatment, unless a child is uncomfortable.

  3. Treatment of fever may mask other signs that would help in the diagnosis.

B. Intervention
1. Provide comfort measures and institute antipyretic actions for temperatures >101° F (38.5° C).
2. Give the child acetaminophen or ibuprofen.
3. Place the child in a cool room, dressed in light pajamas; cover the child only with a sheet (unless the child has chills).
4. Offer cool fluids, and provide cool, moist compresses to the skin.
    a) Tepid sponge baths or hypothermia baths are recommended only for temperatures greater than 104° F (40° C).
    b) Alcohol baths are not recommended for children.
    c) Avoid cooling the child to the point of shivering, because this increases body temperature.

 ALERT: Children should not receive aspirin because of the risk of Reye syndrome, which is associated with the use of aspirin during a febrile viral infection. Since the cause of illness is often unknown in the early stages of fever, it is best to avoid using aspirin in children.

IV. Neutropenia

A. Introduction
1. Neutropenia is a decreased number of neutrophils (absolute neutrophil count [ANC]) with an ANC <1,000 in infants and 1,500 in children.
2. Neutropenia results from a decreased production of or increased destruction of neutrophils.
3. It increases susceptibility to opportunistic infection because the body cannot initiate the immune response.

B. Assessment
1. Be aware that signs of inflammation may be altered (no pus; limited redness and swelling).
2. Assess for irritability and anorexia, which may be the only sign.
3. Note that the WBC count indicates a low ANC, which is the actual number rather than the percentage of neutrophils.
4. The ANC indicates the degree of immune system functioning.
    a) Five hundred to 1,000 indicates moderate risk for infection.

b) Less than 500 indicates a severe risk of life-threatening infection.

5. There are three methods to calculate the ANC:

   a) (Bands + Segs)% × True WBC = ANC

   b) ([Bands + Segs] × WBC)/100 = ANC

   c) (Bands + Segs) × (Abbreviated WBC × 10) = ANC

6. Culture all body orifices to help in early detection of bacterial growth.

C. Interventions

1. Decrease the child's contact with pathogens.

   a) Provide a private room or a roommate without an infection.

   b) Teach proper hand washing.

2. Initiate protective isolation if the ANC is less than 500/mm^3.

3. Provide proper oral hygiene.

4. Provide antibiotics as ordered.

V. Hypogammaglobulinemia

A. Introduction

1. Hypogammaglobulinemia is the absence or deficient production of B cells and antibodies; it may be congenital or acquired.

2. Passive IgG protection from the mother to the child decreases during the first year of life, so symptoms usually appear after age 6 months.

3. The child is susceptible to pyogenic bacterial infections.

B. Assessment

1. Review the child's history for recurrent upper respiratory tract infections, otitis media, skin infections, meningitis, or pneumonia.

2. Assess for signs and symptoms of malabsorption, which may result in immunodeficiency.

C. Interventions

1. Administer monthly gamma globulin injections.

2. Be aware that immunizations may not result in protective antibodies.

VI. Acquired immunodeficiency syndrome (AIDS)/human immunodeficiency virus (HIV) disease

A. Introduction
1. AIDS is an acquired immune deficiency that results from HIV attacking CD4/helper T cells.
2. The majority of children in the United States who contract HIV disease do so in utero or perinatally by being born to an HIV-positive mother; other children with HIV are teens in high-risk categories (sexual contact; sharing contaminated needles) or who have hemophilia and contracted HIV via blood products before universal blood donor screening in 1985.
3. AIDS is not spread by casual contact with an infected child; it is spread only by an exchange of body fluid, including breast milk.

B. Assessment
1. Check for mononucleosis-like prodromal symptoms.
2. Ask about night sweats and recurring diarrhea.
3. Observe for weight loss and failure to thrive.
4. Assess for lymphadenopathy.
5. Note recurrent opportunistic infections (especially lymphoid interstitial pneumonia and *P. carinii* pneumonia), autoimmune disorders, and persistent oral candidiasis, which are common in AIDS.
6. Assess for neurologic impairment, such as loss of motor milestones.

C. Interventions
1. Prevent transmission of HIV.
    a) Promote voluntary HIV testing among all pregnant women in the United States as recommended by the American Academy of Pediatrics; an HIV-positive woman who is treated during pregnancy with zidovudine (AZT) has a decreased risk of giving birth to a child with HIV.
    b) Use standard precautions: wear gloves when handling any bodily secretions.
    c) Wash hands thoroughly.
    d) Use a 10% solution of household bleach in water; applied over 1 minute, to kill HIV outside the body.
    e) Discourage the teenager from engaging in high-risk behaviors; teach safe sex behaviors.

2. Prevent opportunistic and other infections.

a) Administer AZT during early infancy to any infant born to an HIV-positive mother and until the infant's HIV status can be determined (e.g., maternal antibodies are no longer present).

b) Administer co-trimoxazole (Bactrim) prophylaxis to prevent *P. carinii* pneumonia.

c) Administer AZT and other antiretroviral drugs as ordered to the child with low helper T-cell counts.

d) Administer routine childhood immunizations. All vaccines are recommended except varicella because of its live component. MMR is given except in the severely immunocompromised child.

e) Administer gamma globulin monthly because the HIV-positive child does not have an effective T-cell function to drive antibody production.

3. Provide adequate nutrition.

a) Offer high-calorie, high-protein foods including nutritional supplements.

b) Monitor growth and potential for failure to thrive.

4. Provide child and family teaching.

a) Be sure to include the following points in your teaching plan for the parents of a child with HIV:

(1) Hand washing procedures

(2) How and when to use protective equipment, such as gloves, gowns, and masks

(3) Household and laundry cleaning measures

(4) Care of patient's eating utensils

(5) Spill cleanup

(6) Disposal of contaminated equipment and supplies

(7) Trash disposal

VII. Hypersensitivity reactions: Allergies

A. Introduction

1. An allergy is an activation of the immune response by normal environmental antigens.

2. Common allergens include inhalants, dust, insect bites, contactants, foods, animal dander, heat, and cold.

3. Allergic reactions can be immediate or delayed, genetic or acquired.

4. Allergy shots (desensitization) consist of doses of an allergen at levels low enough so that the body does not respond.

         a) Weekly shots of increasing doses can build tolerance.

         b) Not all allergies can be treated in this way.

    5. The exclusively breast-fed infant has a decreased incidence of allergy.

B. Classification of allergies

    1. Type I (immediate hypersensitivity): an IgE-mediated response against the allergen; it is the most common type of allergy

         a) IgE attaches to the mast cell, causing it to release histamine.

         b) Histamine dilates and increases the permeability of vessels resulting in erythema, swelling, and irritation; it also constricts smooth muscles in vascular and bronchiolar tissue resulting in wheezing; it can cause urticaria (hives) and angioedema.

         c) Anaphylaxis can result: hypotension, respiratory distress, "itch all over."

         d) Examples include hay fever, respiratory allergies, and bee stings.

    2. Type II (cytolytic-cytotoxic): the antigen is blood-cell bound

         a) IgM and IgG activate complement.

         b) Examples include transfusion reaction, Rh incompatibility, idiopathic thrombocytopenia purpura, and autoimmune hemolytic anemia.

    3. Type III (immune complex–Arthus reaction): the antigen circulates freely

         a) IgG and IgM respond, and complement damage of the body organs can result.

         b) Examples include systemic lupus erythematosus, rheumatic fever, glomerulonephritis, type 1 diabetes, and rheumatoid arthritis.

    4. Type IV

         a) The reaction occurs in 48 to 72 hours.

         b) Examples include contact dermatitis, poison ivy, PPD reaction, and graft rejection.

C. Respiratory allergies

    1. Introduction

         a) Respiratory allergies are type I allergies that release histamine into the eyes, ears, nose, and throat, resulting in increased vessel permeability and discomfort.

         b) They usually occur in reaction to inhalants (pollen, animal dander, dust, latex), injectants (bee stings), and ingestants.

2. Assessment
   a) Obtain a history of allergies and how and when symptoms occur.
   b) Conduct allergy skin tests to identify the cause.
   c) Note profuse rhinorrhea, nasal obstruction, and bouts of sneezing.
   d) Note allergic shiners (dark circles under the eyes from venous dilation and edema).
   e) Note the allergic salute (pushing up and out on the base of the nose), which will produce a crease across the bridge of the nose.
   f) Note open-mouth breathing, leading to a dry mouth and increasing the risk of respiratory infections.
   g) Check for structural change of the oral cavity and malocclusion.
   h) Note itchy, watery eyes and itching in the back of the throat.
3. Intervention to relieve attacks
   a) Administer antihistamines, bronchodilators (if ordered), and anti-inflammatory agents (if ordered).
   b) Apply cool compresses to the eyes.
   c) Administer vasoconstricting nasal spray.
   d) For anaphylaxis, administer epinephrine via an EpiPen; this constricts blood vessels and relaxes smooth muscles of the respiratory tract; administer right through the clothing into the thigh.
4. Intervention to prevent attacks
   a) Use environmental controls (avoid the allergen; keep the child in an air-conditioned room during grass-cutting or when the pollen count is high).
   b) Permit only damp dusting.
   c) Prevent mold development.
   d) Restrict rugs, stuffed animals, drapes, and natural fibers; use a plastic-wrapped mattress; decrease clutter.
   e) Avoid smoking in the child's environment.
   f) Administer allergy shots (immunotherapy), if appropriate.

D. Gastrointestinal allergies
1. Introduction
   a) The most common allergens include cow's milk, shellfish, nuts (especially peanuts), wheat, citrus, berries, egg whites, chocolate, and pork.

      b)   Food allergy differs from food intolerance conditions, such as celiac disease, lactose intolerance, and Crohn's disease.

2. Assessment
   a) Review the child's history for food types and amounts that cause symptoms.
   b) Ask how soon symptoms occur after ingestion.
   c) Determine which symptoms occur (vomiting, diarrhea, colic, oral skin irritation, respiratory distress).
   d) Observe for failure to thrive.

3. Interventions
   a) Identify the cause, and eliminate it from the child's diet.
   b) Have the child eat the suspected food again after symptoms disappear to see if they reappear (unless the initial reaction caused anaphylaxis).
   c) Be aware that skin tests and allergy shots have not proved beneficial.
   d) Teach family to read labels carefully.
   e) Check environment to make sure that there is no mixing of offending allergen with other products (silverware, cutting surfaces).

E. Dermatologic allergies: Eczema
   1. Introduction
      a) A type I reaction, common in infants, is chronic, with exacerbations and remissions.
      b) Eczema can be caused or aggravated by foods, contactants (especially latex and wool), temperature changes, emotional factors, frequent bathing, and sweating.
   2. Assessment
      a) Observe for red, oozing, highly pruritic vesicles that crust.
      b) Assess for secondary infections and skin thickening from scratching the lesions.
      c) Check for lesions on the cheeks, scalp, wrists, ankles, and antecubital and popliteal areas.
      d) Assess for irritability, fretfulness, and insomnia.
      e) Observe for dry and scaly skin; hard skin cannot trap water.
   3. Interventions to decrease dryness, inflammation, and pruritus
      a) Avoid wool; use lightweight cotton.
      b) Avoid heat and sweatng; keep the child dry.

c) Bathe the child only twice a week, with no soap or very mild soap.

d) Apply topical emollient to the skin immediately after the bath; pat dry.

e) To prevent complications from scratching, keep the nails short; use hand mitts if necessary, and cover affected areas with light clothing.

f) Rinse laundry thoroughly, and use a mild detergent.

g) Administer antihistamines and antibiotics, if ordered.

h) Apply a cortisone cream to decrease inflammation; use a topical lubricating cream on top.

i) Apply cool wet compresses with saline or Burow's solution (aluminum acetate) to decrease itching and make crusts easier to remove.

j) Avoid allergy-triggering foods.

k) Encourage parents to humidify the home during the winter.

VIII. Autoimmune conditions

A. Introduction
1. The immune cells identify self-tissues as foreign antigens and attack them.
2. This produces a loss of self-tolerance.
3. Antibodies attack a self-organ and activate complement, with resulting organ damage.
4. A predisposition to autoimmune conditions may be genetically based in HLA.

B. Examples of autoimmune disease and organs attacked by self-antibodies
1. Acute glomerulonephritis develops in the glomerulus of the kidney.
2. Juvenile rheumatoid arthritis occurs in the synovial lining of joints.
3. Rheumatic fever affects the cardiac muscles and valves.
4. Type I juvenile diabetes affects the islet cells of the pancreas.
5. Multiple sclerosis develops in the myelin.
6. Systemic lupus erythematosus occurs in the DNA of the connective tissue; can result in arthritis, altered kidney function leading to failure, butterfly rash and sun sensitivity, and hematologic and central nervous system disorders.

C. Interventions
   1. Administer immunosuppressant medications such as cortisone to decrease the attack of the immune system against the self.
   2. Implement other interventions specific to each condition.

CHAPTER

8

Cancer

LEARNING OBJECTIVES

1. Assess and plan care for the major types of pediatric cancer.

2. Describe the staging protocols for various solid tumors.

3. Anticipate the psychosocial needs of the child with cancer and the needs of the child's family.

4. Assess the child's perception of death at various stages of development, and plan appropriate interventions when death is imminent.

I. Cancer

A. Overview

1. An alteration in cell function resulting from the overproduction of immature and nonfunctional cells; tissues enlarge for no physiologic function

2. Cause unknown; some types have a genetic basis, as well as the presence of oncogenes; some are related to viruses or to environmental carcinogenic agents; and others have a higher incidence with other conditions (e.g., Down syndrome)

3. Can be life threatening and can metastasize to distant locations

4. Can invade and destroy healthy tissues

5. Goal of treatment is to achieve remission; a 5-year remission is considered a "cure"

B. Pediatric cancers

1. They are second to accidents as the greatest cause of death in children

2. They occur primarily in rapidly differentiating tissues, such as bone marrow

3. Most solid tumors are sarcomas.

4. Cancers in order of frequency in children are leukemia, central nervous system tumors, lymphomas, neuroblastoma, Wilms' tumor, retinoblastoma, rhabdomyosarcoma, and bone tumors.

5. Any tumor in the child is considered malignant until histologically identified, even if it is encapsulated.

6. Childhood cancers grow faster than adult cancers because body tissues are normally in a state of rapid growth and high metabolic rate.

7. The incidence of cancer increases with age.

C. Assessment

1. Be aware that signs and symptoms vary with the type and location of cancer.

2. Assess for pain, abnormal skin lesions, fatigue, fever, and weight loss.

3. Assess for any unusual mass or swelling.

4. Assess for a sudden tendency to bruise.

5. Note any persistent localized pain or limping.

6. Ask about headaches that may be associated with vomiting.

7. Assess for vision changes.

8. Laboratory studies will identify abnormal or immature cells; imaging studies will identify masses; biopsies will identify cancerous cells and assist with staging.

9. Assess for invasion of or pressure on body structures by the tumor.

D. Interventions

1. Be aware that a multifaceted treatment program to prolong survival may include surgery, irradiation, chemotherapy, and occasionally immunotherapy; treatment plans are often based on national cancer protocols.

2. Assist with IV and intrathecal chemotherapy.

   a) Be aware that chemotherapy may include such drugs as cyclophosphamide (Cytoxan), methotrexate, vincristine, and prednisone.

   b) Help the child deal with the side effects of chemotherapy, such as alopecia, vomiting, stomatitis, neurotoxicity, hemorrhagic cystitis, and bone marrow depression.

   c) Initiate measures to prevent the sequelae of chemotherapy.

   (1) Ensure that IV lines are patent, as many drugs cause phlebitis and tissue damage if they escape from the vessel (vesicants/sclerosing agents can cause severe cellular damage if even minute amounts infiltrate into surrounding tissues). Central lines are frequently used and require meticulous sterile care.

   (2) Force fluids to assist in clearing medication from the system.

   (3) Maintain close monitoring of IV medications and infuse slowly.

   (4) Prevent physical contact when mixing chemotherapy drugs, and prepare in a ventilated room.

   (5) For stomatitis, provide a bland, soft diet, use a soft sponge toothbrush, and rinse the mouth frequently with saline or local anesthetic mouthwashes.

   (6) Assist in dealing with any resulting hair loss.

   (7) Take measures to decrease pathogens in the environment; assess the ANC.

   (8) If nausea and vomiting occur, identify foods most palatable (and nutritious) to the child, and provide these whenever the child is able to eat.

d) If child is anemic, oxygen may be needed; if platelets are low, great caution should be taken regarding any invasive treatments.

3. Assist with radiation and help the child deal with its side effects, such as vomiting, alopecia, mucosal ulceration, diarrhea, desquamation of the skin, and myelosuppression.

   a) Administer antiemetics as ordered; provide mouth care.

   b) Provide good skin care, but do not remove skin markings for radiation fields.

4. Prepare for possible biopsy, staging protocols, tumor removal, bone marrow transplantation, organ removal, and palliation.

5. Anticipate after-effects years after treatment, such as genetic changes, learning disabilities, secondary cancers, and altered function of specific organ systems.

6. Use coping strategies(e.g., play therapy, relaxation techniques, and imagery) to deal with the pain and disability.

II. Leukemia

A. Overview

1. Abnormal, uncontrolled proliferation of WBCs

   a) WBCs are producing so rapidly that immature cells (blast cells) are released into the circulation.

   b) Blast cells are nonfunctional, cannot fight infection, and multiply continuously without respect to the body's needs.

   c) Blast cells appear in the peripheral blood, where they normally do not appear.

   d) Blast cells may be as high as 95% in the bone marrow (they are normally less than 5%) as measured by marrow aspiration in the posterior iliac crest (the sternum cannot be used in children).

   e) The increased proliferation of WBCs robs healthy cells of nutrition.

   f) Bone marrow first undergoes hypertrophy, possibly resulting in pathologic fractures.

   g) Bone marrow then undergoes atrophy, resulting in a decrease in all blood cells, which leads to anemia, bleeding disorders, and immunosuppression.

   h) Leukemia is highly associated with ionizing radiation, Down syndrome, chemicals, and virus.

2. Acute lymphoblastic leukemia (ALL)
   a) This is the most common type of leukemia and cancer in children.
   b) Peak age is 2 to 5 years.
   c) Ninety percent to 95% of children with ALL achieve a first remission; almost 80% live 5 years.
   d) The child between ages 3 and 9 with ALL and an initial WBC count of less than 50,000 mm^3 at the time of diagnosis has the best prognosis.
3. Acute myelogenous leukemia (AML)
   a) More common than ALL in adolescents.
   b) Fifty percent to 70% of adolescents with AML reach a first remission; 15% live 5 years.
   c) Death usually follows overwhelming infection.

B. Assessment
   1. Assess for bone pain from hypertrophy of the marrow cavity.
   2. Review the child's history for infections.
   3. Assess for signs and symptoms of anemia.
   4. Observe for petechiae and ecchymosis.
   5. Test urine, sputum, stool, and any emesis for blood.
   6. Ask about nosebleeds, poor wound healing, and oral lesions.
   7. Palpate for lymphadenopathy.
   8. Prepare for lumbar puncture, which indicates whether leukemic cells have crossed the blood-brain barrier.

C. Interventions
   1. Prevent infection; give special attention to mouth care.
   2. Inspect the skin frequently.
   3. Use interventions for anemia and thrombocytopenia.
   4. Give increased fluids to flush chemotherapy through the kidneys.
   5. Provide a high-protein, high-calorie, bland diet.
   6. Provide pain relief.
   7. Monitor the central nervous system for involvement.
   8. Gear nursing measures toward easing the side effects of radiation and chemotherapy.
   9. Help the child and the family allay their fears and guilt.
   10. Offer hope, if appropriate.
   11. Help the child adjust to changes in body image.
   12. Refer parents and adolescents with cancer to support groups.

III. Hodgkin's lymphoma

A. Overview
   1. A malignant neoplasm of the lymphoid tissue
   2. Commonly seen in adolescents and young adults
   3. Usually originates in a localized group of lymph nodes and proliferates via lymphocytes
   4. Excellent prognosis

B. Diagnosis and staging
   1. Methods of making a definite diagnosis
      a) Computed tomographic scan and gallium scan
      b) Lymphangiogram
         (1) Dye is injected intravenously into the feet.
         (2) X-rays track the dye as it travels up the body and is absorbed by the infected nodes.
      c) Lymph nodes and bone marrow biopsies
   2. Stages
      a) In stage I, a single lymph node is involved.
      b) In stage II, two or more lymph nodes on the same side of the diaphragm are involved.
      c) In stage III, nodes on both sides of the diaphragm are involved.
      d) In stage IV, there is diffuse metastasis.
      e) Any stage also designated as "A" exhibits no systemic symptoms; a "B" designation indicates symptoms of fever, night sweats, and weight loss in the preceding 6 months.

C. Assessment
   1. Assess for painless, firm, persistently enlarged lymph nodes that appear insidiously; they are most common in the lower cervical region.
   2. Ask about night sweats and pruritus.
   3. Review the child's or adolescent's history for recurrent fever.
   4. Assess for weight loss.

D. Interventions
   1. Assist with chemotherapy.
   2. Assist with radiation.
   3. Gear nursing measures toward easing the side effects of radiation and chemotherapy.

IV. Non-Hodgkin's lymphoma

   A. Introduction
1. It includes lymphosarcoma, reticulum cell sarcoma, and Burkitt's lymphoma.
2. It metastasizes faster than Hodgkin's.
   - *a)* The primary tumor arises in any lymphoid tissue.
   - *b)* The lymphoma spreads beyond nodes into neighboring tissue.
3. Prognosis for aggressively treated localized disease approaches 90% survival; for those with advanced disease, survival is greater than 75%.

   B. Assessment
1. Assess for enlarged lymph nodes, most common in the lower cervical region.
2. Note that symptoms depend on the organ involved.
3. Assess for night sweats, fatigue, malaise, weight loss, and fever.

   C. Interventions
1. Implement nursing care as for the child with leukemia.
2. Aggressive chemotherapy is implemented.

V. Brain tumors *(see Chapter 14, Central Nervous System Conditions)*

VI. Neuroblastoma

   A. Overview
1. Tumors arise from embryonic cells in the neural crest that give rise to the adrenal medulla and the sympathetic ganglia.
2. Tumors usually arise from the adrenal gland but can also arise at multiple other sites.
3. It is most common in those under age 2.
4. The cancer usually metastasizes before it is diagnosed.
   - *a)* Highly malignant
   - *b)* Poor prognosis (<50%) for the child over age 1; prognosis approaches 75% survival for children diagnosed under age 1 year
5. If a tumor is in the abdomen, it resembles Wilms' tumor.

   B. Diagnosis and staging
1. Methods of making a definite diagnosis
   - *a)* Skeletal scans/computed tomographic scan
   - *b)* Twenty-four-hour urine collection to measure catecholamines, preceded by a vanillylmandelic acid diet for 3 days (eliminate bananas, nuts, chocolate, vanilla)

2. Stages
   a) In stage I, the tumor is confined to the organ or structure of origin.
   b) In stage II, continuity extends beyond the primary site but not across the midline.
   c) In stage III, the tumor extends beyond the midline with bilateral regional lymph node involvement.
   d) In stage IV, the tumor metastasizes.

C. Assessment
   1. Note the location and stage of the tumor, which is usually firm and nontender.
   2. Be aware that the symptoms vary and are often from compression of the tumor on adjacent structures.

D. Interventions
   1. These depend on the location and stage of the tumor.
   2. Chemotherapy is initiated.

VII. Nephroblastoma (Wilms' tumor)

A. Overview
   1. Wilms' tumor is an embryonal cancer of the kidney originating during fetal life.
   2. The average age at diagnosis is 2 to 4 years.
   3. The tumor favors the left kidney and is usually unilateral.
   4. The tumor remains encapsulated for a long time.
   5. The prognosis is excellent if there is no metastasis.

B. Staging
   1. In stage I, the tumor is limited to the kidney.
   2. In stage II, the tumor extends beyond the kidney but can be completely excised.
   3. In stage III, the tumor spreads but is confined to the abdomen and lymph nodes.
   4. In stage IV, the tumor metastasizes to the lung, liver, bone, and brain.

C. Assessment
   1. Assess for a nontender mass, usually midline near the liver; it is often identified by the parent while bathing or dressing the child.
   2. Expect IV pyelography to assess kidney function.
   3. Note any abdominal pain, hypertension, hematuria, anemia, or constipation.

D. Interventions (preoperative)
1. *Do not palpate the abdomen*, and prevent others from doing so; it may disseminate cancer cells to other sites.
2. Handle and bathe the child carefully.
3. Loosen clothing near the abdomen.
4. Prepare the family for a nephrectomy within 24 to 48 hours of diagnosis.

E. Interventions (postoperative)
1. Provide routine care as for a nephrectomy patient.
2. Be aware that chemotherapy and radiation will follow healing.

VIII. Osteogenic sarcoma

A. Overview
1. This is the most common bone cancer in children.
2. Peak age is late adolescence; rare in young children.
3. It usually involves the diaphyseal long bones; about 50% of cases are in the femur.
4. It is highly malignant; metastasizes quickly to the lungs.
5. Survival rate is about 60%.

B. Assessment
1. Note a sunburst effect on the X-ray.
2. Assess pain and swelling at the site.
3. Assess for a history of trauma preceding the pain.
4. Assess for pathologic fractures, which may result from bone marrow involvement.

C. Interventions
1. Reinforce the fact that the child did not cause the tumor.
2. Anticipate amputation at the joint proximal to the tumor; some institutions remove only the bone and salvage the limb.
3. Provide psychological support and reinforcement of the child's strengths.
4. Provide support through phantom limb pain.
5. Provide stump care and help the child prepare for a prosthesis.
6. Assist with chemotherapy.

IX. Ewing's tumor or sarcoma

A. Overview
1. Arises from cells within the bone marrow rather than the osseous tissue
2. Occurs between ages 4 and 25
3. Highly malignant to lungs and bone

B. Assessment
1. Note pain and swelling at the site.
2. Note that the bone has a moth-eaten appearance on the X-ray.

C. Interventions
1. Assist with radiation and chemotherapy.
2. Note that amputation is not routine, since the tumor spreads easily through the bone marrow.

X. Rhabdomyosarcoma

A. Refers to soft tissue sarcomas
1. Muscles, tendons, fibrous connective tissue, vascular tissue
2. Can occur in the orbits, nasopharynx, sinuses, middle ear, abdomen, or perineum

XI. Retinoblastoma

A. Arises from the retina

XII. Graft-versus-host reaction following tissue transplantation

A. Overview
1. A graft-versus-host reaction may occur only if the host is immunologically incompetent; receives live, functioning, and immunologically competent cells; and is genetically different from the host.
2. The graft rejects the entire host.
3. The spleen, lymph nodes, thymus, and bone marrow are rich sources of immunocompetent cells that react against the HLA of nonself antigens.
4. The reaction occurs 10 days to several months after a transplantation, from cell-mediated cytotoxicity.
5. Graft-versus-host reaction primarily affects the liver, GI tract, and skin.

B. Assessment
1. Note increased bilirubin.
2. Assess for diarrhea.
3. Observe for a rash leading to desquamation.

C. Interventions
1. Expect to suppress the rejection with immunosuppressive drugs such as steroids, azathioprine (Imuran), or cyclosporine.
2. Observe for signs of infection; ensure protective isolation.

XIII. Death and dying

A. Language and cognitive development affect perceptions of death.
 1. Give the child facts and elicit the child's feelings; allow the child to hope.
 2. Use language appropriate to the child's cognitive age.
     a) Do not substitute clichés, such as "passed away," for the word "death."
     b) Do not refer to death as sleep; the child may be afraid to go to bed.
 3. The child may seem unresponsive to the information at first; allow time for the information to be processed.

B. Death is viewed differently at different stages of development.
 1. Toddler
     a) Has no concept of time or space other than the here-and-now
     b) Fears death only as an extension of the primary fear of separation from the parents
 2. Preschooler
     a) Perceives death as only a temporary departure
     b) May relate death to sleep
     c) May fear separation from parents; may worry about who will provide care after death
     d) Possesses a rudimentary concept of time
 3. School-age child
     a) Understands the past, present, and future; understands death's permanence
     b) Engages in games that play-act death; perceives death as immobility
     c) Possesses a concrete understanding of causality; may interpret illness as a punishment for a misdeed
     d) Fears pain and abandonment
     e) Is curious about the rituals of death; may ask directly about own death
 4. Adolescent
     a) Expresses anger because of inability to be independent or plan future goals
     b) May want to plan own funeral
     c) May want to complete projects, make tapes to loved ones, or give belongings to others as a way of keeping part of self alive

C. Take the following steps when death is imminent.
   1. Ensure that a parent, relative, or health care person remains with the child at all times to diminish fears of abandonment.
   2. Discuss everyday life events or even death itself; encourage touching and hugging.
   3. Encourage quiet, passive play that provided satisfaction in the past.
   4. Help parents do all that they can do emotionally.
   5. Be aware of the parents' responses to the potential death of their child.
      a) Fear of the unexpected
      b) Anger
      c) Guilt at the thought that they caused the problem by not observing the symptoms earlier, not seeking health care earlier, or not providing a safe environment for their child
   6. Include siblings and grandparents in the dying process.
   7. Involve the chaplaincy department.

CHAPTER
9

Cardiac Conditions

LEARNING OBJECTIVES

1. Differentiate between cyanotic, acyanotic, and obstructive heart defects.
2. Plan care for a child with a cyanotic or acyanotic defect.
3. Plan care for a chilld with an acquired heart condition.

I. Fetal cardiac structures

A. There are three fetal cardiac structures, two of which have significant implications for the newborn.

   1. Ductus venosus is a tube that bypasses the fetus' liver; its purpose is to prevent the rich oxygenated blood from the mother from being diverted to the liver, thus allowing it to be quickly disseminated through the fetus' body; as soon as the umbilical cord is cut, the ductus venosus ceases to function.

   2. Ductus arteriosus is a small fistula between the pulmonary artery and the aorta; the lungs are not yet functioning, and therefore the pressure is higher in the pulmonary artery than in the aorta; the small amount of blood that does go to the right ventricle and up the pulmonary artery is diverted through the ductus arteriosus into the aorta and out to the body.

   3. Foramen ovale is an opening with a one-way flap that allows the blood flowing from the mother through the inferior vena cava into the right atrium to bypass the lungs and proceed directly to the left atrium through this foramen ovale so that the oxygenated blood from the mother can be disseminated through the fetus' body. At birth, with the first breath, there is a pressure change in the heart, and the increased pressure on the left side forces the flap of the foramen ovale to close.

II. Cardiac pressures

A. Pressures on the left side of the heart are higher than on the right side after birth, with the highest internal pressure in the left ventricle.

B. In most cardiac anomalies involving communication between chambers, blood will flow from areas of high pressure to areas of low pressure; this is called a left-to-right shunt.

C. In communicating structures that do not involve chambers, such as patent ductus arteriosus, blood will also flow from high- to low-pressure areas (from aorta to pulmonary artery).

D. Increased flow to the right side causes tissue hypertrophy from increased pressure and increased blood flow to the lungs.

E. The pressure eventually equalizes between chambers as the right side of the heart begins to fail in its attempt to compensate.

F. Contraction of the heart is systole; relaxation of the heart is diastole.

III. Heart rate and blood pressure changes with age

A. Heart rate decreases with age.
   1. Infant: 120-130 beats/min
   2. Toddler/preschooler: 80-105 beats/min
   3. School age: 70-80 beats/min

B. Blood pressure increases with age.
   1. Infant: 80/40 mmHg
   2. Toddler: 80-100/64 mmHg
   3. School age: 94-112/56-60 mmHg

IV. Electrical system of the heart

A. Sinoatrial (SA) node is the heart's pacemaker; it is in the right atrium near where the superior vena cava enters the heart.

B. Charge spreads to atrioventricular (AV) node near the atrial septum near the endocardial cushion (center core of the heart) at the bottom of the right atrium close to the ventricular septum.

C. Charge spreads to bundle of His along the sides of the ventricular septum and then to the Purkinje fibers that stimulate the ventricles to contract.

V. Cyanotic heart defects

A. Introduction
   1. A cyanotic heart defect is a cardiac anomaly in which oxygenated blood entering the aorta and eventual systemic circulation is mixed with deoxygenated blood.
   2. It can result from any condition that increases pulmonary vascular resistance (leading to a right-to-left shunt) or from a structural defect that allows the aorta to receive blood from the right side of the heart.
   3. It can lead to left-sided heart failure, decreased oxygen supply to the body, and the development of collateral circulation.

B. General assessment (for any cyanotic heart defect)
   1. Observe for cyanosis, especially increasing with crying.
   2. Assess for increased pulse and respiratory rates.
   3. Note whether the complete blood cell count shows polycythemia; hypoxia stimulates the body to increase red blood cell production.
   4. Review the child's history for irritability and difficulty with feeding.

5. Observe for clubbing of digits (thickening of fingers and toes because of chronic hypoxemia).
6. Observe whether the child naturally assumes a squatting position; this position increases systemic venous return, shunts blood from the extremities to the head and trunk, and thus decreases cyanosis.
7. Note alterations in blood gas measurements.
8. Assess intake and output; output should be at least 1 to 2 ml/kg/hr (neonates should be 0.5-1 ml/kg/hr).
9. Tests to diagnose and assess cardiac defects include
   a) Electrocardiogram (to evaluate the electrical conduction system, as well as the rate and rhythm)
   b) Cardiac catheterization (to evaluate pressures and oxygen saturations within heart chambers, as well as function of heart)
   c) Echocardiography (uses ultrasound to measure heart size and function)

C. General interventions for any cyanotic heart defect
1. Plan and implement care as you would for a child with anemia (see Chapter 5).
2. Provide oxygen; decrease oxygen demands on the child by anticipating needs and preventing distress.
3. Use a preemie nipple to decrease the energy needed for sucking.
4. Do not interfere when the child is squatting as long as the child appears comfortable; infants may be more comfortable when placed in a knee-chest position.
5. Provide adequate hydration to prevent sequelae of polycythemia.
6. Provide passive stimulation.
7. Administer antibiotics prophylactically to prevent endocarditis.
8. Provide thorough skin care.
9. Prepare the child for cardiac catheterization.
10. Help parents understand the difference between palliative and corrective procedures.

D. Transposition of the great vessels/arteries
1. Introduction
   a) The aorta arises from the right ventricle; the pulmonary artery arises from the left ventricle.

   b) Deoxygenated blood recirculates from the right side of the heart back to the systemic circulation; oxygenated blood recirculates from the lungs to the left side of the heart and back to the lungs.

   c) The child will not survive without communication between these two systems.

  2. Assessment

   a) Note increasing cyanosis as the foramen ovale or ductus arteriosus closes; the foramen may remain open longer because of altered cardiac pressures.

   b) Note other symptoms of a cyanotic heart defect.

  3. Interventions

   a) Prepare the child for cardiac catheterization.

   b) Expect the use of prostaglandin E to keep the ductus arteriosus open.

   c) Prepare the child for possible palliative surgery to provide communication between the right and left chambers.

   d) Prepare the child for possible corrective surgery in first weeks of life (arterial switch procedure).

E. Tetralogy of Fallot

  1. Introduction

   a) The defect consists of pulmonary artery stenosis, ventricular septal defect (VSD), hypertrophy of the right ventricle, and an overriding aorta (dextroposition of the aorta—the placement of the aorta is closer to the ventricular septum).

   b) The aorta sits over the VSD and receives blood from the right and left ventricles.

   c) Pulmonic stenosis reduces blood flow to the lungs; blood with a low oxygen concentration exits into the systemic circulation.

   d) The condition stems from increased pressure in the right ventricle; blood shunts right to left, forcing deoxygenated blood to the left side and up the aorta.

  2. Assessment

   a) Observe for cyanosis.

   b) Note polycythemia.

   c) Observe for posturing, such as squatting or the knee-chest position.

   d) Note dyspnea, clubbing of digits, failure to thrive, exercise intolerance, and other symptoms of cyanotic heart disease.

       e) Be aware that the infant may have episodes of increasing cyanosis and hypoxia of blood going to the brain, leading to short periods of loss of consciousness ("tet spells").

   3. Interventions

       a) Prepare the child for cardiac catheterization.

       b) Prepare for complete repair during the first year or palliative treatment to increase blood flow to the lungs.

       c) Administer morphine during a tet spell to decrease infundibular spasm.

       d) Begin other interventions as for cyanotic heart defects.

F. Hypoplastic left heart syndromes

   1. Introduction

       a) Hypoplastic left heart syndrome consists of aortic valve atresia, mitral atresia or stenosis, a diminutive or absent left ventricle, and severe hypoplasia of the ascending aorta and aortic arch.

       b) In this condition, blood from the left atrium travels through an atrial septal defect or patent foramen ovale (left-to-right shunt) to the right ventricle and pulmonary artery, entering the system via the ductus arteriosus.

   2. Assessment

       a) Assess for increasing dyspnea, cyanosis, and tachypnea during the first few days after birth; without treatment, congestive heart failure (CHF) develops as the ductus closes.

       b) Remember that the child may appear normal at birth.

   3. Interventions

       a) Prepare the child for cardiac catheterization.

       b) Expect the use of prostaglandin E to keep the ductus arteriosus patent.

       c) Prepare the child for surgical interventions (Norwood procedure), which allows the use of the right atrium as a pumping chamber for pulmonary circulation and the right ventricle as a systemic pumping chamber; if available, the child may receive a heart transplant.

       d) Be aware that death will occur in early infancy without surgery, although the mortality rate is 25% with surgery.

VI. Acyanotic heart defects

A. Introduction
   1. Blood entering the aorta is completely oxygenated.
   2. Acyanotic heart defects include those in the septa that result in a left-to-right shunt (any increased blood volume on the right side of the heart causes right-sided hypertrophy and increased blood flow to the lungs) and those between structures that inhibit blood flow to the system or after pulmonary resistance.
   3. Such a defect can result in cyanosis if the right side of the heart fails or not enough oxygenated blood enters the circulation.
   4. CHF is frequently seen secondary to a congenital heart defect in which structural abnormalities result in an increased volume load or increased pressure load on the ventricles. Any anomaly resulting in increased blood flow to the lungs, such as conditions resulting in a left-to-right shunt, can cause CHF. Clinical manifestations vary among children, but early symptoms are tachycardia, diaphoresis, tachypnea, fatigue, and mild cyanosis. Early recognition and treatment of CHF lessens the impact on long-term growth and development.

B. General assessment (for any acyanotic heart defect)
   1. Assess for respiratory distress, congested cough, and diaphoresis, which may indicate congestive heart failure from increased blood flow to the lungs.
   2. Note increases in pulse and respiratory rates to compensate for increased blood flow to the lungs; assess vital signs.
   3. Check for hepatomegaly; blood has difficulty entering the right side of the heart and backs up in the liver.
   4. Review the child's history for frequent respiratory infections from increased pulmonary secretions.
   5. Assess for poor growth and development from increased energy expenditure for breathing.
   6. Evaluate the degree of fatigue.
   7. Assess for a heart murmur.

C. General interventions (for any acyanotic heart defect)
   1. Expect to administer digoxin to decrease the pulse rate and strengthen cardiac contractions (bradycardia is a pulse of less than 100 beats/min in infants); take apical pulse for 1 minute before administration; order must specify minimum heart rate for administration.

    2. Monitor fluid status.
       a) Administer a diuretic, such as furosemide (Lasix), and observe for potassium loss.
       b) Enforce fluid restrictions.
       c) Monitor fluid intake and output, weigh soiled diapers; weigh the child daily.
    3. Reduce oxygen demands by organizing physical care and anticipating the child's needs.
    4. Give the child high-calorie foods that are easy to ingest and digest.
    5. Prevent cold stress by maintaining a normal body temperature.
    6. Prevent infection; administer antibiotics prophylactically to prevent endocarditis.
    7. Prepare the child for cardiac catheterization.

  D. Patent ductus arteriosus (PDA)
    1. Introduction
       a) PDA results from failure of the fetal structure to close; it is common in premature infants.
       b) PDA leads to the shunting of blood to the pulmonary artery (because pressure in the aorta is higher than in the pulmonary artery), which increases blood flow to the lungs.
    2. Assessment
       a) Be aware that the child may be asymptomatic except for a machinelike heart murmur.
       b) Assess for signs and symptoms of CHF and left ventricular hypertrophy.
    3. Interventions
       a) Prepare the child for cardiac catheterization.
       b) Prepare for possible administration of the prostaglandin inhibitor indomethacin to achieve pharmacologic closure.
       c) Prepare for possible surgical correction, which involves ligating the PDA in a closed-heart operation.

  E. Ventricular septal defect (VSD)
    1. Introduction
       a) VSD is the most common congenital cardiac anomaly.
       b) It occurs when a septum fails to complete its formation between the ventricles, resulting in a left-to-right shunt.
    2. Assessment
       a) Assess for signs and symptoms of CHF with right ventricular hypertrophy.

   b) Assess for failure to thrive.

   c) Evaluate the degree of fatigue.

   d) Review the child's history for recurrent respiratory infections.

  3. Interventions

   a) Prepare the child for cardiac catheterization.

   b) Prepare for possible pulmonary artery banding to prevent CHF; a permanent correction with a patch is performed later, when the heart is larger.

    (1) Be aware that closure of a VSD may interfere with the electrical conduction of the heart, leading to heart block.

   c) Be aware that some children experience spontaneous closure of the VSD by age 3.

 F. Atrial septal defect (ASD)

  1. Introduction

   a) ASD stems from a patent foramen ovale or the failure of a septum to develop completely between the atria.

   b) It results in a left-to-right shunt.

   c) It may resolve spontaneously by age 5.

  2. Assessment

   a) Assess for signs and symptoms of CHF.

   b) Be aware that the child may be asymptomatic except for a heart murmur.

  3. Interventions

   a) Prepare the child for cardiac catheterization.

   b) Mild defects may close spontaneously.

   c) Prepare the child for surgical correction, which involves patching the hole; some ASDs can be corrected during a cardiac catheterization.

VII. Obstructive defects

 A. Pulmonic stenosis

  1. Introduction

   a) Pulmonic stenosis involves a narrowing or fusing of the valves at the entrance of the pulmonary artery interfering with right ventricular outflow.

   b) It may result in right ventricular hypertrophy and right-sided heart failure.

  2. Assessment

   a) Review the child's history for exertional fatigue.

b) Ask about chest pain with exercise, which occurs in mild to moderate pulmonic stenosis.

c) Ask about cyanosis with exercise, which occurs in severe pulmonic stenosis.

d) Auscultate for a systolic murmur.

3. Interventions

a) Prepare the child for cardiac catheterization.

b) Prepare the child for open-heart surgery to separate the pulmonary valve leaflets; this will leave the child with a permanent residual murmur.

B. Aortic stenosis

1. Introduction

a) Aortic stenosis involves a narrowing or fusion of the aortic valves, interfering with left ventricular outflow.

b) It may cause left ventricular hypertrophy, left-sided heart failure, and pulmonary congestion.

2. Assessment

a) Ask about syncope and dizziness.

b) Review the child's history for angina.

c) Ask if activities increase symptoms.

d) Find out which measures bring relief.

3. Interventions

a) Prepare the child for cardiac catheterization to assess the degree of aortic stenosis.

b) Prepare the child for surgical palliation with a valvulotomy or commissurotomy (however, this does not prevent stenosis from recurring in adulthood).

C. Coarctation of the aorta

1. Introduction

a) Coarctation of the aorta involves a narrowing of the aortic arch, usually distal to the ductus arteriosus beyond the left subclavian artery.

b) It decreases blood flow to the trunk and lower extremities and increases blood flow to the head and arms.

c) The condition predisposes the child to a cerebrovascular accident (stroke).

2. Assessment

a) Assess for full bounding pulses in the arms and weak or absent pulses in the legs, but the same pulse rate in both areas.

b) Review the child's history for nosebleeds, headaches, dizziness, leg cramps, and lack of energy.

c) Assess for increased blood pressure in the arms and decreased blood pressure in the legs.

d) Palpate for a warm upper body and a cool lower body.

e) Assess for signs and symptoms of CHF from backup pressure to the left side of the heart.

3. Interventions

a) Prepare the child for cardiac catheterization.

b) Understand that surgery for a coarctation distal to the ductus arteriosus may involve closed-heart resection of the coarcted portion; this is usually not performed until late preschool age.

VIII. Rheumatic fever (RF)

A. Introduction

1. RF is an acquired autoimmune immune-complex disorder occurring 1 to 6 weeks after a group A beta-hemolytic streptococcal infection, in many cases after strep throat that is not treated with penicillin.

a) The streptococcal infection *is not* present in the heart.

b) With an untreated strep infection, RF develops in 1% to 5% of patients.

2. The disorder is caused by the production of antibodies against the toxin of the streptococci; these antibodies attack the heart valves because of similarities in their antigenic markers.

3. RF results in antigen-antibody complexes that initiate complement formation and heart destruction.

4. According to the American Heart Association (AHA), one major and two minor symptoms are needed for diagnosis (known as the Jones criteria).

B. Assessment

1. Use the Jones criteria when assessing for major manifestations: carditis, polyarthritis, chorea, subcutaneous nodules, and erythema marginatum (temporary disk-shaped nonpruritic reddened macules that fade in the center leaving raised margins).

a) Aschoff bodies (fibrinlike plaques) form on the heart valves causing edema and inflammation, resulting in stenosis and leakage of valves.

       b)   Chorea is sudden irregular movements of the extremities that are involuntary and increase with stress.

   2.   Use the Jones criteria when assessing for minor manifestations: history of RF, fever, arthralgia, increased erythrocyte sedimentation rate, altered electrocardiogram with a prolonged P-R interval, and evidence of a strep infection (elevated antistreptolysin-O [ASO] titer).

  C. Interventions

   1.   Administer penicillin to prevent additional damage from future attacks (the child takes it until at least age 20 or for 10 years after the attack, whichever is longer).

   2.   Provide bed rest until the sedimentation rate normalizes.

   3.   Administer anti-inflammatory medication for arthritis pain.

   4.   Institute safety measures for chorea; keep the environment calm, reduce stimulation, avoid the use of forks or glass, assist in walking.

   5.   Maintain growth and development with appropriate passive stimulation.

   6.   Provide emotional support for long-term convalescence.

   7.   Prevent reinfection.

IX. Kawasaki syndrome

  A. Introduction

   1.   Kawasaki syndrome results in vasculitis of the small and medium-sized blood vessels; coronary arteries are most at risk.

   2.   It is the leading cause of acquired heart disease in children.

   3.   Without treatment, about 25% will suffer permanent cardiac sequelae (damage to coronary arteries or damage to heart muscle).

   4.   In the majority of cases, patients are under 5 years of age.

   5.   Etiology is unknown; not transmitted person-to-person.

  B. Assessment

   1.   Assess for high, persistent fever for 5 days with

      a)   Swelling of the conjunctivae without drainage

      b)   Inflammation of the mouth, lips, tongue (strawberry tongue)

      c)   Rash that varies from child to child

      d)   Swollen, red hands and feet

      e)   Cervical lymphadenopathy

     2. Evaluate for signs and symptoms of myocardial infarction (abdominal pain, vomiting, restlessness, irritability without ability to console, pallor).

     3. Assess for signs of fluid overload and CHF.

C. Interventions

     1. Administer immune globulin (IVIG) intravenously to reduce incidence of coronary artery abnormalities, especially when given within 10 days of infection/symptoms.

       a) Side effects include anaphylaxis, headache.

     2. Administer salicylates (aspirin).

       a) First, it is given in an anti-inflammatory dose, and then it is lowered to an antiplatelet dose.

     3. Administer fluids judiciously.

     4. Minimize skin discomfort; provide mouth care and cool cloths or baths.

X. Subacute bacterial endocarditis

A. Introduction

     1. An infection of the valves and inner lining of the heart, it usually affects the mitral or aortic valves (bacterial organisms enter the bloodstream from a site of localized infection and grow in the heart, usually on an area of abnormal blood flow or turbulence).

     2. Those at risk include anyone with a prosthetic device in the heart and anyone with abnormal blood flow in the heart, especially due to congenital cardiac anomalies.

     3. Other risk factors include bacteremia from dental procedures, gum disease, and urinary tract infection.

B. Assessment

     1. Fever

     2. Fatigue

     3. Weight loss

     4. Pallor

     5. New or changes to an existing heart murmur

C. Interventions

     1. IV antibiotics for 6 weeks

     2. Prevention in those who are at high risk

       a) Oral antibiotics prior to any invasive procedure (especially dental) and antibiotics afterwards

XI. Diagnostic tests

A. Cardiac catheterization

1. Prepare the child by using doll play and hospital play; stress the familiar but show where the catheter is inserted and make a security object (blanket, stuffed animal) available.

2. Describe the sensations the child will experience.

3. Establish baseline data before the procedure.

   a) Weigh the child.

   b) Check the child's color, pulse rate, blood pressure, and temperature of extremities.

   c) Check the child's activity level.

4. Keep the affected extremity immobile after catheterization to prevent hemorrhage; observe the dressing for bleeding or hematoma formation; if bleeding occurs, apply direct pressure.

5. Monitor after catheterization; check vital signs, including the intensity of the pulse, and the color and temperature of the extremities; compare all four extremities; compare data with precatheterization baseline data; observe for bleeding or hematoma formation at site.

6. Ensure adequate intake (IV or oral) because of blood loss during the procedure and diuretic action of some dyes used.

XII. Cardiopulmonary pulmonary resuscitation (CPR) guidelines

A. Overview

1. The AHA Guidelines for CPR are categorized according to the age of the victim and the classification of the rescuer. This content is limited to the health care provider rescuer.

B. Unresponsive infant or child

1. Overview

   a) Infant: 0 to 12 months

   b) Child: 1 year to 12-14 years (onset of puberty). Note: The AHA guidelines support the use of pediatric advanced life support guidelines (PALS) to pediatric patients of all ages (usually up to 16-18 years) rather than at the onset of puberty.

2. Sequence

   a) Lone health care provider—witnessing sudden collapse of an infant or child

(1) Call 911 and obtain an automated external defibrillator (AED).

(2) Start CPR and use the AED as follows:

    (*a*) There is no recommendation for or against the use of AEDs for infants <1 year.

    (*b*) For children 1 to 8 years, use a pediatric dose-attenuating system designed to deliver a reduced shock.

b) Lone health care provider—rescuing an unresponsive infant or child.

(1) Open airway and check for breathing.

(2) If no breathing detected, give two rescue breaths.

(3) Check pulse.

    (*a*) Infant: assess brachial pulse.

    (*b*) Child: assess carotid pulse.

(4) If a pulse is detected, perform rescue breaths at a rate of 12 to 20 breaths/min for the infant and child.

(5) If no pulse is detected, perform 5 cycles of compressions to ventilations (30:2). Note: The 30:2 compressions to ventilations is the standard for all age groups for lone-rescuer CPR; the ratio for two-rescuer infant and child CPR is 15:2.

c) If child remains unconscious, leave the victim to call 911 and obtain an AED for use as described above.

3. Rescue breaths

    a) Deliver breath in 1 second; note visible rise of the chest.

    b) If chest does not rise, reopen the airway and reattempt rescue breath.

4. Chest compressions

    a) Location

        (1) Infant: use two fingers just below the nipple line.

        (2) Child: use one hand or two hands as needed.

    b) Depth: compress the chest of the infant or child one third of the chest depth.

5. Rate: compressions should be at a rate of 100 compressions per minute. Note: CPR guidelines changed in 2005. Certification examination questions may reflect previous guidelines below:

C. Sequence for infants and children (0 to 8 years)

1. If you are not alone: direct a bystander to call 911.

2. If you are alone: provide 1 minute of CPR before calling 911.

D. Infant and child CPR guidelines
   1. Rescue breathing: 1 breath every 3 seconds
   2. Chest compressions: 100/minute
   3. Ratio of breaths to compressions: 1:5

CHAPTER
10

Respiratory Conditions

LEARNING OBJECTIVES

1. Describe assessments for respiratory distress in a child.

2. Describe the conditions or complications related to immature lung development in the child.

3. Explain the treatments most commonly implemented for respiratory conditions.

4. Differentiate among various childhood respiratory conditions, and plan appropriate nursing interventions.

I. Developmental perspectives

A. The lungs are not fully developed at birth.

B. The alveoli continue to develop and increase in size through puberty.

C. The child's respiratory tract has a narrower lumen than an adult's until age 5; the narrow airway makes the young child prone to airway obstruction and respiratory distress from inflammation.

D. Respiratory distress results in retractions as other muscles assist with breathing.

E. It is normal for infants to have slightly irregular breathing patterns.

F. Young infants are obligatory nose breathers; they do not tolerate nasal congestion well.

G. Infants and young children have increased susceptibility to ear infections because of eustachian tubes that are shorter, broader, and more horizontally positioned.

H. Ventilation is the movement of gases from the atmosphere into (inspiration) and out of (expiration) the lungs.

I. Diffusion is the movement of inhaled gases in the alveoli and across the alveolar capillary membrane.

J. Perfusion is movement of oxygenated blood from the lungs to the tissues.

II. Respiratory distress

A. Assessment
1. Observe child's face for signs of anxiety.
2. Assess for irritability, combativeness, or decreased responsiveness.
3. Observe the position the child maintains to ease respiratory effort (usually sits up or slightly hyperextends the neck into "sniffing" position).
4. Evaluate the energy and effort needed for the child to breathe; note feeding problems (increased respiratory effort results in fatigue and decreased ability to coordinate suck/ swallow and breathe).
5. Assess respiratory quantity and quality.
   a) Tachypnea = fast respiratory rate (>60/min for newborn).
   b) Hyperpnea = deep respirations.

      c)   Apnea = unintentional cessation in spontaneous breathing for >20 seconds with or without bradycardia and color change.

6. Assess symmetry of chest movement.

7. Assess for change in chest configuration to accommodate increased air trapping (barrel chest) or for congenital chest deformities that interfere with adequate respiratory effort (pigeon chest, pectus excavatum).

8. Assess for nasal flaring (nares widen on inhalation). Assess for open-mouth breathing and chin lag (chin lowers with inhalation).

9. Assess for use of accessory muscles: the child strains the upper neck muscles with inhalation (tracheal tugging) and uses the lower muscles (below rib cage).

      a)   Assess for retractions: suprasternal (directly above sternum), intercostal (between ribs), substernal (below xiphoid process).

10. Assess for finger and toe clubbing (proliferation of terminal phalangeal tissue) from chronic hypoxia.

11. Assess for changes in skin color, such as mottling, pallor, or cyanosis (especially circumoral cyanosis).

12. Assess cardiac tolerance of respiratory alteration.

13. Monitor pulse oximetry (arterial hemoglobin saturation).

14. Measure respiratory capacity using pulmonary function tests (these may not be accurate because the young child has trouble following directions); these measure lung volumes and lung function.

15. Evaluate chest X-rays (ensure adequate protection by covering the child's gonads and thyroid gland with a lead apron).

16. Monitor blood gas measurements.

      a)   Assess for hypercapnia (excessive CO_2 in the blood because of inability to blow off CO_2).

      b)   Assess for hypoxia (decreased tissue oxygenation).

          (1) Increase in partial pressure of arterial CO_2 stimulates ventilation.

          (2) Decrease in arterial CO_2 inhibits ventilation.

17. Peak flow measurement is an estimate of the greatest flow velocity during a forced expiration.

18. Auscultate the lungs for absent or diminished breath sounds and adventitious sounds (inspiratory or expiratory wheeze [a whistling noise as air is forced through a narrow passage]): crackles (rales), rhonchi, and wheezes.

19. Assess for expiratory grunting, which is an attempt to increase end expiratory pressure and prolong the exchange of oxygen and CO_2; common with chest pain, pulmonary edema, and respiratory distress syndrome (RDS).
20. Assess for inspiratory stridor (a harsh sound from laryngeal or tracheal edema while trying to inhale).
21. Assess for a hoarse cough or muffled speech.
22. Assess for a cough and note whether it is dry or congested, paroxysmal or intermittent, productive or nonproductive (a cough is productive if the child coughs up mucus and swallows it; mucus need not be expectorated for a cough to be considered productive).
23. Percuss for dullness, which indicates that air has been replaced by fluid or solid tissue.

B. Interventions
1. Administer oxygen (oxygen tent, Oxyhood, blow-by oxygen, nasal cannula/prongs); the need is guided by pulse oxygenation and clinical assessments; the route is guided by patient age and developmental level.
   a) When using an oxygen tent
      (1) Keep plastic sides down and tucked in, because oxygen is heavier than air, so the loss is greater at the bottom of the tent.
      (2) Keep plastic away from the child's face.
      (3) Prevent the use of toys that produce sparks or friction.
      (4) Frequently assess oxygen concentration.
      (5) To return child to a tent that has been opened, put tent sides down, turn on oxygen, wait until the oxygen is at the prescribed concentration, and then place the child in the tent.
      (6) Check temperature inside tent, as tent may become warm; if cooling mechanism is used, check child to ensure that the child is warm and not suffering from cold stress; if mist is used, change clothing and bedding often to keep child dry.
      (7) Comfort child and assure the child that he/she will not be left alone in the tent.
      (8) Remember that oxygen is a drug and can cause damage to lung tissue if given in high doses.

     b)   For use of nasal cannulas

        (1) Remove nasal secretions from end of tubing frequently.

        (2) Administer saline nose drops to moisten passages.

2. Perform chest physiotherapy, percussion, and postural drainage.

     a)   These loosen secretions and enhance expectoration via gravity.

     b)   Perform at least 30 minutes before meals.

     c)   Use a cupped hand over a covered rib cage for 2 to 5 minutes on the five major positions (upper anterior lobes, upper posterior lobes, lower posterior lobes, and right and left sides) for a maximum of 20 to 30 minutes; for infants, preformed rubber percussors are available.

     d)   Administer aerosol-nebulized medications immediately before percussion and postural drainage.

3. Perform nasal suctioning using a bulb syringe or nasotracheal suction using low pressure.

4. Use saline solution nose drops to relieve nasal stuffiness.

     a)   Teach the parents how to prepare this solution at home by mixing 1/8 teaspoon salt in 4 oz sterile water.

     b)   Administer 1 or 2 drops in each nostril, and use a bulb suction if needed.

5. Teach the child breathing exercises to enhance aeration and increase respiratory muscle tone.

     a)   Teach exercises to expand the chest (deep breathing), to compress the chest (sit-ups or toe-touching), and to increase respiratory efficiency (jumping jacks).

     b)   Make each exercise into a game (for example, "Simon says, touch your toes").

     c)   Do not let the child overdo exercises to the point of fatigue.

6. Teach the parents how to use an apnea monitor at home (usually involves the application of one to three leads and how to set alarms).

     a)   Although the monitor helps reassure the parents, the sound of the alarm may frighten them.

     b)   Teach the parents how to assess the child and the machine when the alarm sounds.

7. Organize activities to include rest periods.

8. Elevate the head of the bed to take pressure off the abdominal organs and diaphragm.

9. Avoid oral feedings if the child has tachypnea (respiratory rate >60/min) or dyspnea to prevent aspiration.

   a) If the child is in mild distress, encourage small, frequent, slow feedings of clear liquids to prevent aspiration.

   b) Avoid milk (it tends to promote phlegm production).

10. Expect to give antihistamines if symptoms stem from allergy; these medications are not given for the common cold or for cystic fibrosis, because they dry up secretions, countering measures aimed at liquefying them.

11. Expect to administer decongestants.

12. Expect to administer antitussives for a dry cough; do not try to suppress a productive cough because the mucus will block the airway.

13. Teach the parents to shield the child from respiratory irritants, such as baby powder and cigarette smoke.

14. Do not hyperextend the young child's neck, as it will decrease the diameter of the airway.

15. Keep the environment calm.

16. If tracheostomy tubes are in place, only insert suction catheter to no more than 0.5 cm beyond the end of the trach tube; do *not* insert until obstruction is felt, as this will cause trauma to the tracheobronchial wall.

   a) Do *not* routinely instill saline solution before suctioning unless ordered; this contributes to bacterial colonization and decreases arterial oxygen saturation (Sao_2).

III. Upper respiratory tract infections (nasopharyngitis)

A. Introduction

1. Only the upper airway is involved.

2. Nasal blockage interferes with infant feeding (the infant is an obligate nose breather).

3. Rhinorrhea may be serous or mucopurulent.

4. The child normally has 6 to 9 colds per year.

B. Assessment

1. Assess the degree of respiratory distress.

2. Check the child's temperature.

3. Check the throat for white lesions, and take a culture if appropriate.

    4. Differentiate a cold from a respiratory allergy by history (see Table 2).
    5. Assess behavioral changes.
  C. Interventions
    1. Take measures to reduce fever.
    2. Provide decongestants and a vaporizer, and encourage rest and increased fluid intake.
    3. Use saline nose drops and gentle suction with a bulb syringe in the infant, especially before feeding.
    4. Ensure adequate fluid intake.
    5. Administer antibiotics if a bacterial cause is suspected.

Table 2. Differentiating respiratory allergies from the common cold

Allergies	Common cold
Usually *not* accompanied by fever	Fever may or may not be present
Usually occur in a seasonal pattern	No pattern
May constantly sneeze	Sneezing may be sporadic
Presence of allergic shiners and nasal crease; mucus is usually clear and watery	Mucus may be purulent, yellow, or green; allergic shiners and nasal crease usually not present
Pruritus of the nasal passage, back of throat, and inner ear	May be accompanied by sore throat; usually *not* accompanied by pruritus of eyes and nose
Family history of allergies	History of contagion among friends and family
Eosinophils present in nasal smear	Eosinophils absent in nasal smear

IV. Tonsillitis

  A. Introduction
    1. Tonsils are lymph organs guarding the entrance to the respiratory and gastrointestinal (GI) systems.
    2. Tonsils should not be removed unless they occlude the airway, have atrophied and no longer function, or are chronically infected.
    3. Tonsillitis can be treated with antibiotics at home; tonsillectomy requires prehospitalization preparation of the child for a same-day or overnight procedure.

B. Assessment
   1. Review the child's history of allergy symptoms to differentiate from bacterial tonsillitis.
   2. Assess for signs of ear infection and upper respiratory tract infection.
   3. Assess respiratory effort.
   4. Inspect the child's mouth for loose teeth.

C. Interventions (preoperative)
   1. Explain sights and sounds of operating room (OR)/short procedure unit.
   2. Reinforce that the child will be in a "special sleep" so the child will not feel the procedure.
   3. Allow child to play with equipment (stethoscope, sphygmomanometer).
   4. Assure child that he/she will never be alone and encourage parents to stay at bedside.
   5. Put child's special blanket/animal/toy in the recovery area for child (label it to avoid loss).
   6. Prepare child for a sore throat and a way to communicate the degree to which the throat hurts.

D. Interventions (postoperative)
   1. Place child in a prone or side-lying position to facilitate drainage.
   2. Do not suction except in a respiratory emergency; suction will cause trauma to the site and possible hemorrhage.
   3. Check for frequent swallowing, pallor, restlessness, a fast thready pulse, or vomiting bright red blood (these are signs of hemorrhage and require immediate attention). Vomiting of dark dried blood is common.
   4. Provide an ice collar for comfort and for reducing edema.
   5. Provide clear, cool, noncitrus fluids (do not offer red fluids, which can be mistaken for blood if vomited). Do not use straw to avoid damaging sutures.
   6. Discourage from activities that may irritate surgical site (coughing, blowing nose, clearing throat).
   7. Inform parents that
      a) Bleeding is most likely to occur in the first 24 hours or 7 to 10 days after tonsillectomy.
      b) The back of the throat will look white and have an odor for the first 7 to 8 days after surgery; this is not a sign of infection.

V. Otitis media (middle ear infection)

A. Introduction
1. It is common in infants because ear canal is shorter, wider, and less angled.
2. This is a common complication of upper respiratory tract infections; it is caused by blockage of the eustachian tubes (blockage results in unequal pressure between the middle ear and the outside environment and possible introduction of a virus or bacteria into the middle ear).

B. Assessment
1. Assess for a bulging, red tympanic membrane.
2. Assess for pain; note that the infant pulls on or rubs the ear when in pain.
3. Observe for irritability.
4. Assess for signs and symptoms of upper respiratory tract infection.
5. Note the degree of fever.

C. Interventions
1. Administer antibiotics orally or as ear drops, if ordered.
   a) Remember to pull the earlobe down and back when administering eardrops to infants.
2. Administer analgesics and antipyretics.
3. Administer decongestants to relieve eustachian tube obstruction.
4. (For chronic otitis media.) Be aware that a myringotomy may be performed to drain the middle ear and equalize pressure (tubes are inserted into the tympanic membrane; it is common for them to fall out).
   a) Postoperatively, position on affected side to facilitate drainage.
   b) Instruct parents to keep ear canal clean and dry; keep water out of ears.
5. Prevent some cases by feeding infants in upright position and administering pneumococcal vaccine.

VI. Epiglottitis

A. Introduction
1. A potentially life-threatening infection of the epiglottis, most commonly affecting children ages 2 to 6
2. Most common causative organism is bacterial *Haemophilus influenzae*

       3.   Incidence decreased significantly since the introduction of the Hib vaccine

B. Assessment

     1.   Assess for difficult and painful swallowing; note increased drooling, refusal to drink, and stridor.

     2.   Listen for muffled, hoarse, or absent speech.

     3.   Note fever, irritability, and restlessness.

     4.   Note tachycardia and tachypnea; the child may extend the neck in a sniffing position.

     5.   Ask about a sore throat.

C. Interventions

     1.   Defer inspecting the throat; inspection of the throat could stimulate a spasm of the epiglottis and cause respiratory occlusion.

     2.   Have equipment ready for a tracheotomy and intubation.

     3.   Decrease number of personnel examining child to decrease child's anxiety; allow child to sit on parent's lap (the sitting position makes breathing easier).

     4.   Administer antibiotics, as ordered.

VII. Croup (acute spasmodic laryngitis; acute laryngotracheobronchitis)

A. Introduction

     1.   Croup commonly affects toddlers

     2.   It is usually viral-induced edema of the larynx, which results in the "seal bark" cough.

     3.   Symptoms usually begin at night and during cold weather.

     4.   Condition can recur.

B. Assessment

     1.   Note a barking, brassy cough or hoarseness.

     2.   Note inspiratory stridor with varying degrees of respiratory distress.

     3.   Assess for increased dyspnea and lower accessory muscle use; rales and decreased breath sounds indicate that the condition has progressed to the bronchi.

C. Intervention (for care of the child at home)

     1.   Keep child calm to ease respiratory effort and conserve energy.

     2.   Use cool-air vaporizer (or mist tents in the hospital).[Some recommend taking the child outside for a few minutes to breathe in the cool night air, or standing in front of the open freezer; this should decrease laryngeal spasm (do not let the child become chilled)].

3. Child may vomit large amounts of mucus; this vomiting does not require medical treatment.
4. Encourage clear liquid intake to keep hydrated.
5. Inform parent of signs of respiratory distress that would require hospitalization.

VIII. Bronchiolitis: Obstruction of the small airways (bronchioles)

A. Introduction
   1. This is a lower airway infection characterized by thick mucus.
   2. It typically affects infants younger than 6 months of age; most common in the winter and spring.
   3. Most common organism is respiratory syncytial virus (RSV).
      a) Other causes are parainfluenza and adenovirus.
   4. Mortality rate for infants with RSV is 1% to 6%.
   5. It is spread by respiratory contact with secretions; spread by direct contact, not airborne droplets; spreads up to 3 feet when coughed or on hands and clothes of providers.
      a) It can survive for hours on surfaces and for 30 minutes on the skin.
   6. RSV is prevented in high-risk infants by monthly doses of RSV-IVIG or RespiGam; this provides sensitized antibodies against RSV; palivizumab (Synagis) may be given prophylactically to decrease the severity of the condition.

B. Assessment
   1. X-ray shows hyperinflation (because of air trapping) and patchy atelectasis (collapsing of end airways).
   2. Assess for RSV nasal aspirate for inpatients.
   3. Anticipate thick mucus and signs of respiratory distress.

C. Interventions
   1. Elevate head of bed.
   2. Provide humidified oxygen (humidifier is controversial).
   3. Expect to administer IV fluids.
   4. Aspirate nasal secretions before feeding, if feeding is allowed.
   5. Administer small frequent feedings.
   6. Administer nebulized albuterol (this is best practice, but findings are nonconclusive).
   7. Use gloves, gowns, and hand washing as secretion precautions.
   8. Administer chest physiotherapy after edema has abated.

IX. Asthma (reactive airway disease)

A. Introduction

1. Chronic reversible obstructive inflammatory airway disease, caused by an increased reaction (hypersensitivity) of the airways to various stimuli, especially allergens, exercise, or irritants (chemicals, perfumes, smoke) or a change in the weather; may also be idiopathic

2. Classic symptoms: bronchoconstriction (of smooth muscle), chronic inflammation of the airways, increased mucus production, all leading to airway obstruction and air trapping

3. Chronic condition with exacerbations

B. Assessment

1. Evaluate degree of respiratory distress: dyspnea, use of accessory muscles, unequal or decreased breath sounds; crackles.

2. Auscultate for prolonged expiration with an expiratory wheeze; in severe distress, an inspiratory wheeze may be heard.

3. Evaluate oxygen saturation via pulse oximetry and blood gas measurement; they may show increased $Paco_2$ from respiratory acidosis.

4. Assess the nature of the child's cough.

   a) Ask about a history of a cough at night (often a first sign).

   b) Is cough hacking, nonproductive, productive?

5. Child may complain of chest tightness (or stomach hurting).

6. Observe for an alteration in chest contour (barrel chest) from chronic air trapping.

7. Assess neurologic state (severe hypoxia can alter cerebral function).

8. Note fatigue and apprehension; assess for emotional stress.

9. Rule out respiratory infection.

10. Assess for a positive family history of allergies; assess for environmental and home allergens.

11. Review child's history for exercise intolerance.

12. Keep twice daily (b.i.d.) records of peak expiratory flow rates within 15 minutes of medication administration.

C. Intervention (to prevent an attack)

1. Administer skin tests to identify sources of allergy; begin hyposensitization through the use of allergy shots, if applicable.

2. Modify the environment to avoid an allergic reaction; remove the offending allergen.
3. Administer long term controller medications, (see Table 3) such as:
    a) Cromolyn sodium.
        (1) It prevents release of mast cell products after an antigen-IgE reaction.
        (2) Rinse child's mouth after inhalation of medication to prevent oral thrush.
    b) Inhaled corticosteroids
    c) Leukotriene Modifiers (Anti-inflammatory)
        (1) Montelukast (Singulair)
        (2) Zafirlukast (Accolate)
        (3) Zileuton (Zyflo)
    d) Long Acting Inhaled Beta-2 Agonists
        (1) Salmeterol
4. For exercise-induced asthma, give prophylactic treatments 10 to 15 minutes before exercise (e.g., cromolyn sodium or β-adrenergic agents).
5. Many medications are administered through nebulizers; this allows medication to be deposited in the lungs and avoids systemic reactions to the medications.
    a) Have child take slow, deep breaths through the mouth; this avoids particles being deposited in the nose and pharynx.
6. Preventive medications usually administered with a metered dose inhaler (MDI) with a spacer attached (the medication can be puffed into the spacer/holding chamber by the child and then inhaled; this avoids the problem of coordinating the activities of pressing the MDI and inhaling slowly).
7. Teach breathing exercises to increase ventilatory capacity.
8. Recommend against smoking in the child's environment.
9. For chronic asthma, administer daily doses of inhaled corticosteroid to control chronic inflammation.

D. Interventions during an asthma attack
1. Allow child to sit upright to ease breathing; provide moist oxygen, if necessary.
2. Administer bronchodilator (e.g., β-agonist [albuterol]), and oral corticosteroid (short course), as ordered.
    a) Side effects of bronchodilators include increased heart rate, nervousness, vomiting, headache, tremors, sleeplessness.

    b) Side effects from other asthma medications include increased heart rate, stomach ache, dry mouth, hoarseness, sore throat, thrush.

   3. Administer IV fluids to keep mucus moist.

   4. Maintain a calm environment; provide emotional support and reassurance.

   5. Failure to respond to medications to ease bronchoconstriction is called status asthmaticus and requires an emergency response.

Table 3. Common asthma medications

Drug category	Examples	Comments
Short-acting inhaled β_2-agonists	Albuterol (Proventil, Ventolin)	Bronchodilators
Inhaled corticosteroids	Beclomethasone (Vanceril), budesonide (Pulmicort), fluticasone (Flovent, Advair), triamcinolone (Azmacort)	Anti-inflammatory for long term use
Oral corticosteroids	Prednisolone, Methylprednisolone, Prednisone	Short term anti-inflammatory
Preventive	Cromolyn (Intal) and nedocromil (Tilade)	Prevents IgE from binding with allergen
Leukotriene modifiers	Montelukast (Singulair), zafirlukast (Accolade)	Anti-inflammatory
Anticholinergics	Iperatropian bromide (Atrovent)	Bronchodilators

X. Cystic fibrosis (CF)

 A. Introduction

   1. CF is an inherited autosomal recessive disease of the exocrine glands; involves a faulty gene on chromosome 7 (delta 508 resulting in the CF transmembrane regulator protein).

   2. It is the most common genetic disease in the United States in Whites.

   3. Death is almost always caused by respiratory compromise; portal hypertension related to cirrhosis of the liver can result in esophageal varices; average age of life span is mid 30s.

4. Most patients have little or no release of pancreatic enzymes (lipase, amylase, and trypsin).
5. Exocrine organs are obstructed by the increased and constant production of mucus.
   a) Onset of secondary diabetes increases in incidence as children with CF approach adulthood.
6. The child sweats normally, but the sweat contains 2 to 5 times the normal levels of sodium and chloride.
   a) This is the basis for the diagnostic pilocarpine iontophoresis sweat test (and why parents used to describe their child as "tasting salty").
   b) Therefore, salt depletion may occur during hot weather and heavy exercise.
7. DNA testing for CF is mandated in some states for newborns.
8. Males are sterile from blockage or absence of the vas deferens; females have increased mucus in their reproductive tract, making conception difficult but possible.

B. Assessment
   1. Gastrointestinal
      a) Assess for meconium ileus in the newborn (blockage of small intestines at or near the ileo-cecal valve from a lack of pancreatic enzymes); seen in 7% to 10% of newborns with CF.
      b) Assess stools for steatorrhea (excessive stool fat, bulky, greasy, foul-smelling, and contain undigested food).
      c) Assess for failure to thrive because of malabsorption.
      d) Observe for distended abdomen and thin arms and legs.
      e) Assess appetite (child may have a voracious appetite, although the body is unable to absorb many of the nutrients ingested).
      f) Assess for rectal prolapse.
   2. Respiratory
      a) Assess for degree of respiratory distress.
      b) Assess quality of the chronic cough and the mucus; is it worse than it normally is? Is the mucus more viscous and a different color?
      c) Assess for oxygenation status (pulse oximetry, skin color, clubbing of digits).
      d) Assess for signs of respiratory infection.
      e) Assess for signs of chronic obstructive respiratory disease (barrel chest related to air trapping).
      f) Assess for sinusitis and nasal polyps.

C. Interventions

1. Administer pancreatic enzymes *with* meals and snacks.

2. Provide high-calorie, high-protein foods with added salt; infants may need predigested formula, such as Pregestimil; may require enteral feedings at night to provide necessary caloric intake.

3. Give multivitamins, especially A, D, E, and K (fat-soluble vitamins) in a water-miscible form.

4. Perform pulmonary hygiene (chest percussion, postural drainage, and vibration [percussion will release mucus from bronchial walls; postural drainage uses gravity to allow mucus to be expectorated]) 2 to 4 times per day preceded by mucolytic, bronchodilator, or antibiotic nebulizer inhalation treatment.

   a) Use a cupped hand over a covered rib cage for 2 to 5 minutes on each area of the lung (upper anterior lobes, upper posterior lobes, lower posterior lobes, right and left sides).

   b) Avoid doing percussion during periods of acute bronchoconstriction or airway edema (as during an asthma attack or croup) to prevent mucus plugs from loosening and causing airway obstruction; avoid when pulmonary hemorrhage is present. Do not put in the "head-down" position if increased intracranial pressure exists.

   c) Flutter mucus clearance device is a tube one blows into that assists in increasing sputum expectoration.

   d) ThAIRapy vest provides high-frequency chest wall vibrations to help loosen secretions.

   e) Aerosolized Pulmozyme (recombinant human deoxyribonuclease [DNase]) decreases viscosity of mucus.

      (1) Inhaled DNAse is used to thin mucus before chest physiotherapy.

5. Treat infection promptly and aggressively because bacterial colonization leads to progressive destruction of lung tissue; *Pseudomonas aeruginosa* (difficult to eradicate), *Burkholderia cepacia* (increases morbidity and mortality), and *Staphylococcus aureus* are most common.

6. Treat diabetes once it is diagnosed.

7. Encourage to be physically active, alternating with rest periods.

8. Teach parents to avoid administering cough suppressants and antihistamines; the child must be able to cough and expectorate to prevent pulmonary obstruction.
9. Promote annual immunization for influenza.
10. Initiate genetic counseling for the family and for the adolescent with CF.
11. Promote as normal a life as possible.
12. As teens with CF reach adulthood, they may require assistance with reproduction and also may require a lung transplant.

XI. Respiratory distress syndrome (RDS)

A. Introduction
   1. Commonly seen in premature infant because of underdeveloped lungs and uninflated alveoli in the absence of surfactant

B. Assessment
   1. Observe for increasing respiratory distress, grunting respirations, and increased respiratory rate.
   2. Note whether child's X-ray has a ground-glass appearance; assess for atelectasis.
   3. Note whether the child requires increased energy to breathe, which may result in exhaustion.
   4. Monitor for abnormal blood gas measurements that may signal hypoxia.

C. Interventions
   1. Expect the child to be receiving continuous positive airway pressure (CPAP) if case is mild or mechanical ventilation to keep alveoli open.
   2. Administer surfactant within first 24 hours.
   3. Organize care to ensure minimal handling.
   4. Control child's temperature to reduce stress and decrease additional energy use.
   5. Use aseptic technique to reduce the risk of infection.
   6. Administer IV fluids to ensure adequate hydration, but withhold food and fluids because of the child's high respiratory rate; anticipate possible nasogastric (NG) tube feedings.
   7. Turn child every 2 hours; raise head of bed; provide developmental care; enhance bonding between parents and child.
   8. Perform chest physiotherapy before suctioning.

XII. Bronchopulmonary dysplasia (BPD)

A. Introduction
1. BPD is a complication of RDS resulting from high oxygen concentration and long-term assisted ventilation.
2. Epithelial damage occurs with the thickening and fibrotic proliferation of the alveolar walls and damage to the bronchiolar epithelium.
3. Ciliary activity is inhibited, so the child has trouble clearing mucus from the lungs.
4. Recovery usually occurs in 6 to 12 months; however, the child may remain ventilator or oxygen dependent for years.

B. Assessment
1. Be aware that the child may have no symptoms initially.
2. Assess for oxygen and ventilator dependency; monitor for dyspnea and hypoxia without this assistance.

C. Interventions
1. Oxygen, by cannula, tracheostomy, or ventilator is often required; remember that oxygen is a medication (room air is 21% oxygen).
2. Because of increased airway resistance, bronchodilators are administered.
3. Dexamethasone therapy may be given to reduce inflammation.
4. Diuretics may be given, because of a tendency to accumulate interstitial fluid in the lung.
5. Administer chest physiotherapy.
6. Increased oxygen consumption results in a higher need for calories without increasing the amount of fluid.
7. Promote normal development; for children using ventilators, teach sign language so that the child can communicate with you.
8. Provide adequate time for rest.

XIII. Foreign body aspiration

A. Introduction
1. It is common in infants and toddlers.
   a) Airways are narrow.
   b) Curiosity is high.
2. It usually involves food, toys, or environmental agents.
3. Dried bean aspiration poses greatest danger because beans absorb respiratory moisture and swell, forming an obstruction; peanuts cause an immediate emphysema reaction.

      4.   Most objects end up in right bronchus because it is straighter and wider than left.

B. Assessment
1. Assess for respiratory distress.
2. Examine mouth and throat to locate foreign body.
3. Be aware that the object may be expelled spontaneously.

C. Intervention
1. If airway is occluded, perform abdominal thrust; for infants, back blows and chest thrusts are used to relieve obstruction and to prevent injury to abdominal organs.
2. Assist with measures to open the airway, such as tracheotomy or intubation, if necessary.
3. Assist with bronchoscopy, if necessary.

XIV. Sudden infant death syndrome (SIDS)

A. Introduction
1. SIDS is the sudden death of an infant in which a postmortem examination fails to confirm the cause of death.
2. Peak age is 3 months; 90% occur before age 6 months, especially during winter and early spring months.
3. Death usually occurs during sleep without noise or struggle.
4. Autopsy findings indicate pulmonary edema, intrathoracic petechiae, and other minor changes suggesting hypoxia.
5. The "Back to Sleep" campaign, in which parents are encouraged to place their children on their backs to sleep, has significantly decreased the incidence of SIDS.

B. Interventions (with parents)
1. Provide family with a room and a staff member to stay with them; support them and reinforce the fact that the death was *not* their fault.
2. Prepare the family for how the infant will look and feel.
3. Let parents touch, hold, and rock the infant, if desired; allow them to say good-bye to the infant.
4. Prepare the parents for the need for an autopsy, which is the only way to diagnose SIDS.
5. Have pictures taken of the infant for the family.
6. Contact spiritual advisers, significant others, support systems, and the local SIDS organization.

CHAPTER
11

Renal and Genitourinary Conditions/ Fluid and Electrolyte Balance

LEARNING OBJECTIVES

1. Describe how a child's fluid and electrolyte status differs from that of an adult.

2. Assess and plan care for a dehydrated child.

3. Assess and plan care for a child with infected or inflamed renal and urinary systems.

4. Discuss congenital anomalies of the genitourinary tract.

I. Functions of kidneys

A. Detoxify blood

B. Eliminate wastes

C. Produce erythropoietin in response to hypoxia to stimulate bone marrow to make more RBCs

D. Regulate blood pressure by producing renin
   1. Renin stimulates the production of angiotensin I, which stimulates production of angiotensin II, which causes peripheral vasoconstriction and secretion of aldosterone.
   2. Aldosterone promotes reabsorption of sodium and water and raises blood pressure; aldosterone also increases renal excretion.

E. Maintain fluid and electrolyte balance

F. Regulate acid/base balance

II. Fluid and electrolyte balance

A. Body water and body weight
   1. Water is the body's primary fluid.
   2. The amount varies with age, sex, and percentage of body fat.
      a) The premature infant's weight is 90% water; the term infant's weight is 75% to 80% water.
         (1) The infant has a much greater percentage of total body water in extracellular fluid (42%- 45%) than the adult does (20%).
         (2) The infant therefore cannot conserve water as well as the adult and has less fluid reserve.
      b) Because of the increased percentage of water in a child's extracellular fluid, the child's water turnover rate is 2 to 3 times higher than the adult's; 50% of the infant's extracellular fluid is exchanged every day, compared with only 20% of the adult's.
      c) The child is therefore more susceptible than the adult to dehydration.
      d) The proportion of body water to body weight decreases with increasing age as body fat increases and solid body structures grow.
      e) The distribution of body water does not reach adult levels until late school age.

f) The adult percentage of body water (63% for men, 52% for women) is attained by age 3; after puberty, females have more fat than males and therefore less water weight.

B. Metabolism
1. The child's growth depends on, and results in, an increased metabolic rate.
   a) The child's metabolic rate is 2 to 3 times higher than that of the adult.
   b) The child therefore also produces more metabolic waste.
2. The child's pulse, respiratory, and peristaltic rates are higher than the adult's.
   a) The child has a greater proportion of insensible water loss.
   b) The child therefore needs more water per kilogram of body weight than the adult.

C. Body surface area
1. The newborn has a greater ratio of body surface area to body weight than the adult; this results in greater fluid loss through the skin.
2. Shivering and sweating mechanisms after infancy partially control body temperature.

D. Electrolytes
1. Sodium
   a) Principal cation of extracellular fluid
   b) Influences distribution of body water (water follows sodium) and osmolality
2. Potassium
   a) Principal cation of intracellular fluid
   b) Major determinant of cell membrane resting potential, influencing neuromuscular excitability; too much or too little will negatively affect cardiac conduction
3. Calcium
   a) Helps maintain normal cell membrane permeability
   b) Deficit results in tetany; excess causes hypotonia
   c) A component of bone and teeth and of the clotting cascade
4. Phosphorus
   a) Crucial for energy production for metabolism and growth
   b) Interacts with calcium to promote bone growth
5. Magnesium
   a) Important for muscle and nerve activity

E. Renal function

1. The child attains the adult number of nephrons by age 1 year, although these structures continue to mature throughout early childhood.

2. The infant's renal function can maintain healthy fluid and electrolyte status; however, it does not compensate as efficiently during stress as the adult's.

3. The infant has a low glomerular filtration rate; however, the rate approaches the adult level by age 2.

4. The infant does not concentrate urine at an adult level.

   a) Average specific gravity for the infant is less than 1.010 (water is 1.000).

   b) Average specific gravity for an adult is 1.010 to 1.030.

5. Although the number of daily voidings decreases with increasing age (because of increased urine concentration and better control), the total amount of urine produced daily may not vary significantly; the amount of urine is measured by weighing the diaper and subtracting dry weight from wet weight (grams equals milliliters because of the low specific gravity).

   a) The infant usually voids 5 to 10 ml/hr.

   b) The 4-year-old's bladder holds 250 ml, allowing the child to stay dry through the night.

   c) The 10-year-old usually voids 10 to 25 ml/hr.

   d) The adult usually voids 35 ml/hr.

6. Inefficient reabsorption of sodium can result in hyponatremia.

7. The child has a short urethra.

   a) Organisms can be easily transmitted into the bladder.

   b) The female urethra is closer to the rectum than the male's, posing a greater risk of contamination by incorrect wiping after a bowel movement.

F. Urinary function studies

1. Urine is checked for blood, protein, glucose, ketones, and pH via a dipstick; these substances do not usually spill into the urine and are an indication that more assessment is necessary.

2. Specific gravity also is checked (urine can be collected from the cotton matting in an infant's diaper).

3. Use the clean-catch method to collect urine from an infant.

   a) After properly cleaning the skin and genitals, apply a pediatric urine collector to dry skin (powders and creams should not be used).

4. An IV pyelogram aids in checking renal pelvic structures by X-ray following injection of a contrast material (when describing the procedure to children, refer to the injected dye as "special medicine").

5. A voiding cystourethrogram aids in viewing the bladder and related structures during voiding, especially to detect strictures and reflux.

   a) Contrast material is instilled in the bladder through a catheter.

   b) The young child cannot retain the fluid through sphincter control.

   c) The older child may be frightened or embarrassed by being asked to urinate on the X-ray table.

6. Blood urea nitrogen (BUN) level, creatinine level, and glomerular filtration rate are also evaluated.

   a) Creatinine clearance is the best measure of kidney function; it is the end product of energy metabolism from muscle and so is relatively constant.

      (1) Normal serum creatinine levels for the child are 0.2 to 2.0 mg/dl with variability based on age.

   b) BUN is an index of the glomerular filtration rate.

   c) Glomerular filtration rate measures the amount of plasma from which a given substance is cleared in 1 minute.

G. Maintenance fluid requirements

1. Maintenance fluid requirements are the water and electrolytes required to sustain the expenditure of normal physiologic activities.

2. Maintenance fluid requirements are appropriate for use in term infants >2 weeks of age.

3. The Holliday-Segar method of calculating maintenance fluids is as follows:

Long version for # ml/day

Child's weight in kg:	Multiply by -- ml/day	= Subtotal
1st 10 kg (0-10 kg)	100	A
2nd 10 kg (11-20 kg)	50	B
Each additional kg (>20 kg)	20	C
TOTAL		A + B + C = X ml/day
		(equivalent to the daily maintenance fluid requirement)

Short version for # ml/hr

Child's weight in kg	Multiply by -- ml/hr	= Subtotal
1st 10 kg (0-10 kg)	4	A
2nd 10 kg (11-20 kg)	2	B
Each additional kg (>20 kg)	1	C
TOTAL		A + B + C = X ml/hr
		(equivalent to the hourly maintenance fluid requirement)

Examples:

Child weighs 7 kg (7 kg × 4ml/hr = 28 ml/hr)

Child weighs 15 kg (first 10 kg = 40 ml [10 × 4 ml/hr]; next 5 kg × 2 ml/hr = 10 ml; 40 + 10 = 50 ml/hr)

Child weighs 28 kg (40 ml for first 10 kg; 20 ml for next 10 kg; 8 kg × 1 ml/hr = 8 ml; 40 + 20 + 8 = 68 ml/hr)

H. Dehydration
   1. Introduction
      a) Dehydration can occur from significantly decreased fluid intake or from loss of water and electrolytes via vomiting, diarrhea, or diaphoresis; in dehydration, fluid output usually exceeds intake.
      b) Expressed as a percentage of body weight lost as water, dehydration can be severe enough to produce volume depletion, circulatory collapse, and shock.
      c) Isotonic dehydration is a deficiency of fluid and electrolytes in approximately equal proportions with a normal serum sodium (Na) of 130 to 150 mEq/L.
         (1) Fifteen percent isotonic dehydration in the infant is considered severe.
         (2) Nine percent loss in the older child is considered severe.
      d) In hypotonic dehydration, electrolyte loss is greater than fluid loss with a decreased serum Na <130 mEq/L, causing extracellular-to-intracellular movement of water that results in shock.
      e) In hypertonic dehydration, fluid loss is greater than electrolyte loss with a serum Na >150 mEq/L, causing intracellular-to-extracellular movement of water that results in neurologic changes, such as confusion, inability to concentrate, and motor tremors.

2. Assessment
   a) Assess the quality and quantity of fluid intake and output.
      (1) Intake may be greater than output but insufficient to meet the body's needs.
      (2) Water may be lost in stool or vomiting.
   b) Note decreased urine output and concentrated urine.
   c) Note a sudden weight loss.
   d) Assess for dry skin with poor tissue turgor; assess for a sunken fontanel in the infant.
   e) Assess for a decrease in tears and saliva, dry mucous membranes, sunken and soft eyeballs, and thirst.
   f) Note pale cool skin with poor perfusion, cool extremities, decreased body temperature, tachycardia, tachypnea, and hypotension.
   g) Note lethargy, irritability, and a high-pitched, weak cry.
   h) Note feeding behavior to identify when vomiting or diarrhea occurs in relation to meals, if anorexia exists, or if the child feeds vigorously after vomiting.
3. Interventions
   a) Record hourly all stools, vomitus, and urine.
      (1) Note the amount, color, consistency, concentration, time, and relation to meals or stress.
      (2) Note the results of specific gravity and other values from urine dipstick tests.
   b) Promote fluid intake.
   c) Provide mouth care with lemon and glycerin swabs.
   d) Provide skin care; turn the child every 2 hours and keep the extremities warm.
   e) Measure intake and output carefully.
      (1) Weigh diapers and record fluids used to take medications.
      (2) Indicate the fluid lost by diaphoresis, suctioning, or other tubes.
   f) Weigh the child using the same scale at the same time each day, with the child naked or wearing the same amount of clothing.
   g) Provide rest.
   h) Monitor for and prevent shock.
   i) Withhold food and fluids if vomiting and use IV replacement of fluids; provide sucking stimulation to the young infant.

   j) When restarting fluids for the infant, provide a fluid replacement solution, such as Pedialyte.

   k) When restarting fluids for the older child, begin with flat noncaffeinated soda; do not give solutions with a high sodium content, such as milk or broth (caffeine is a bladder irritant).

   l) Note that any increase in ambient heat or water loss requires greater fluid intake to meet hydration needs.

I. Acid-base balance

 1. Acid-base balance is regulated by the renal, respiratory, and hematologic systems through the regulation of HCO_3 (base) and $PaCO_2$ (acid) to determine serum pH through regulation of H^+.

 2. Important values to consider when assessing acid-base balance are:

  a) Normal serum pH for the child is 7.35 to 7.45.

   (1) pH<7.35 is acidosis (net loss of HCO_3 or gain of H^+)

   (2) pH >7.45 is alkalosis (net gain of HCO_3 or loss of H^+)

  b) Normal serum HCO_3 for the child is 22 mEq/L.

  c) Normal PaO_2 for the child is 96 mmHg.

  d) Normal serum $PaCO_2$ for the child is 37 mmHg.

 3. Always look at the pH first to determine if it is normal.

  a) If the pH is normal, the child's body has compensated for the altered acid-base.

  b) If the pH is abnormal, the acid-base balance is uncompensated.

 4. Disturbances in acid-base balance can be pulmonary or metabolic in origin.

  a) Acidosis is the decrease in the normal physiologic pH.

   (1) Respiratory acidosis is reflected by an increase in $PaCO_2$.

    (a) Respiratory arrest will cause a build up of CO_2 in the blood, since the person is not "blowing it off."

   (2) Metabolic acidosis is reflected by a decrease in HCO_3.

    (a) Increased acid ingestion (as in aspirin poisoning), increased acid production (as in diabetic ketoacidosis), or decreased production of bicarbonate by the kidney (as in kidney failure).

  b) Alkalosis is an increase in the normal physiologic pH.

   (1) Respiratory alkalosis is reflected by a decreased $PaCO_2$, as seen in hyperventilation.

(2) Metabolic alkalosis is reflected by an increase in HCO_3, as seen in increased production of bicarbonate by the kidneys.

5. Aspirin poisoning: An example of metabolic acidosis
    a) Aspirin (acetylsalicylic acid) is an analgesic, antipyretic, and anti-inflammatory agent that inhibits platelet aggregation.
    b) The normal dose is 1 grain per year of age, up to age 10; toxicity occurs at 200 mg/kg.
    c) The body compensates for increased carbonic acid production by increasing the respiratory rate to blow off the excess CO_2.
    d) Assessment
        (1) Observe for an increased respiratory rate from metabolic acidosis.
        (2) Note fever from stimulation of carbohydrate metabolism.
        (3) Note decreased blood glucose levels.
        (4) Note altered clotting function; assess for petechiae and blood loss.
        (5) Check for irritability, restlessness, and tinnitus or altered hearing.
    e) Interventions
        (1) Maintain a patent airway; encourage hyperventilation.
        (2) Perform gastric lavage.
        (3) Ensure adequate hydration to flush the aspirin through the kidneys.

III. Urinary tract infection (UTI)

A. Introduction
    1. A microbial invasion of the urinary tract, UTI is more common in females because of the placement and size of the urethra.
        a) Bladder infection = cystitis
        b) Urethra infection = urethritis
        c) Kidney infection = pyelonephritis
    2. UTI also may be caused by reflux, irritation by bubble baths, poor hygiene, or incomplete bladder emptying.

B. Assessment
    1. Assess the quantity, quality, and frequency of voiding.

2. Note that a clean-catch urine culture will yield large amounts of bacteria.
3. Assess for hematuria and increased urine pH.
4. Ask about a frequent urge to void with pain or burning on urination.
5. Note low-grade fever, lethargy, and poor feeding patterns.
6. Ask about abdominal pain.
7. Assess for enuresis.
8. Assess toileting habits for proper front-to-back wiping and proper hand washing.
9. Assess bathing habits for tub baths or bubble baths.
10. Assess the number of urinary infections per year; UTIs may recur.

C. Interventions
1. Administer an antibiotic, such as sulfonamides (Bactrim/Septra), amoxicillin, nitrofurantoin (Macrodantin), or cephalosporins to prevent glomerulonephritis.
2. Force fluids to flush the infection from the urinary tract (100 ml/kg/day); clear fluids are best; avoid carbonated or caffeinated drinks and chocolate, as they can irritate the bladder mucosa.
3. Teach proper toileting hygiene; encourage the child to use the toilet every 2 hours.
4. Discourage the use of tub baths and bubble baths.
5. Be aware that some children have vesicoureteral reflux, where the urine enters the bladder, only to reflux back up the ureters to the kidney, potentially causing inflammation of both the ureters and the kidney.

IV. Enuresis

A. Introduction
1. Repeated involuntary urination after age 5 is called enuresis; it usually occurs while the child is asleep but also may occur during the day.
2. In primary enuresis, the child has never achieved complete bladder control.
3. In secondary enuresis, the child has achieved a period of bladder control.
4. Suggested causes include stress, incomplete muscle maturation of the bladder, altered sleep patterns, and an irritable bladder that cannot handle large amounts of urine.

B. Assessment
  1. Review the child's history for age of toilet training, onset of enuresis, and frequency of occurrences.
  2. Ask about a history of previous UTIs, burning on urination, and a sense of urgency.
  3. Expect urinalysis, urine culture and sensitivity, and blood studies, including BUN and creatinine to evaluate for UTI and for kidney function.

C. Interventions
  1. Be aware that treatment varies with the cause.
  2. Remind the child to use the toilet every 2 hours.
  3. Decrease fluids after 5 p.m. except to satisfy the child's thirst.
  4. Administer imipramine (Tofranil) to inhibit urination or desmopressin (DDAVP) nasal spray to decrease nighttime urine output, if ordered.
  5. Teach bladder-stretching exercises (retention control training) during the day.
    a) Have the child drink large amounts of fluid.
    b) Try to have the child keep the bladder enlarged for a while before emptying.
  6. Have parent wake child before parent goes to bed and take to bathroom.
  7. Provide emotional support to the child and parents.
    a) Do not embarrass or punish the child.
    b) Do not refer to enuresis as an accident, because accidents can be prevented.
    c) Have child assist in changing sheets.

V. Nephrotic syndrome/nephrosis

A. Introduction
  1. Nephrotic syndrome is an autoimmune process that occurs 1 week after an immune assault; may be idiopathic.
  2. It increases glomerular permeability to protein, especially albumin.
    a) Protein loss results in decreased colloidal osmotic pressure, thus letting fluid escape from intravascular space to interstitial space resulting in edema.
  3. The condition is common among toddlers.
  4. Condition may be self-limiting.

B. Assessment
1. Note proteinuria and hypoproteinemia (hypoalbuminemia).
2. Assess for signs and symptoms of hypovolemia.
3. Note that morning urine will usually have a high protein level.
    a) The urine is dark, foamy, and frothy.
    b) The urine has a high specific gravity.
    c) Urine production decreases.
4. Note that only microscopic hematuria will be manifested; frank bleeding does not occur.
5. Assess for edema.
    a) Dependent body edema accompanies weight gain.
    b) Periorbital edema occurs in the morning.
    c) Abdominal ascites and increased abdominal girth are also evident.
    d) Scrotal edema occurs.
    e) Ankle edema develops by midday.
    f) Diarrhea, anorexia, and malnutrition result from edema of the intestinal mucosa.
    g) Generalized edema = anasarca.
6. Check electrolyte levels, because potassium is lost in the urine with diuresis.
7. Observe for stretched, shiny skin with a waxy pallor.
8. Be aware of increased susceptibility to infection from increased interstitial fluid.
9. Note fatigue or lethargy.
10. Note any anorexia or abdominal pain.
11. Prepare the child for a renal biopsy to diagnose the disease.

C. Interventions
1. Provide skin care to edematous skin; do not use adhesive strip bandages, tape, or intramuscular injections.
2. Provide warm soaks to decrease periorbital edema; elevate the head of the bed.
3. Turn the child frequently; provide scrotal support and place padding between body parts to prevent irritation.
4. Test the first void of the day for protein.
5. Feed small, frequent, high-calorie, high-protein meals without added salt; measure intake, output, and daily weight.
6. Administer corticosteroids to suppress the autoimmune response and to stimulate vascular reabsorption of edema.
7. Prevent contact with persons who have an infection; some immunoglobulins are lost resulting in alterations in immune function.

8. Anticipate diuresis in 1 to 3 weeks.
    a) Maintain bed rest during rapid diuresis.
    b) Monitor hydration status and vital signs.

VI. Acute glomerulonephritis (AGN)

A. Introduction
   1. AGN is an autoimmune immune-complex disorder occurring 1 to 2 weeks after a group A β-hemolytic streptococcal infection.
      a) Antibodies are made against the toxin of the streptococci but attack the glomerulus because of similarities in their antigenic markers.
      b) The condition results in antigen-antibody complexes that initiate the complement reaction and cause renal damage in the glomeruli.
      c) Streptococcus is not present in the kidney at any time.
      d) AGN can also be caused by other organisms, such as pneumococci and viruses.
   2. The disorder is common in children ages 4 to 7 years.

B. Assessment
   1. Assess for signs and symptoms of altered renal function from edema and kidney damage.
   2. Test urine for hematuria; the urine is cola colored (smoky).
   3. Note decreased urine output.
   4. Note results of blood tests.
      a) An increased sedimentation rate indicates inflammation.
      b) An increased antistreptolysin O (ASO) titer indicates a recent streptococcus infection.
   5. Assess for and monitor increased blood pressure.
   6. Note the appearance of periorbital or dependent edema.
   7. Note irritability, lethargy, and an anemic appearance.

C. Interventions
   1. Implement the same measures as for nephrosis.
   2. Monitor intake, output, and daily weight.
   3. Teach the parents about possible antibiotic therapy.
   4. Institute moderate sodium restrictions for the child with hypertension or edema.
   5. Administer medications to control hypertension.

VII. Hemolytic uremic syndrome

A. Introduction
1. Etiology unknown, although it is associated with a recent bacterial or viral infection
2. Most common cause of renal failure in those <3 years of age
3. Includes a triad of symptoms: acute renal failure, hemolytic anemia, and thrombocytopenia
4. Prognosis good, but there may be residual renal impairment

B. Assessment
1. Prodromal symptoms may be respiratory or gastrointestinal (vomiting and diarrhea that may be bloody).
2. Five to 10 days later, pallor, bruising, purpura, oliguria, and irritability may develop.
    a) Measure intake and output.
    b) Assess for flank pain.
    c) Assess skin at least twice daily for new bruising or purpura.
    d) Check urine and stool for blood and protein.
    e) Assess for hypertension.
    f) Weigh daily.
3. Assess for cardiac compensation.

C. Interventions
1. Prepare for dialysis, if ordered.
2. Replace fluid/electrolytes/nutritional needs, but be prepared for fluid restrictions.
3. Handle gently to avoid further bruising.

VIII. Acute renal failure

A. Introduction
1. Multiple causes can result in failure of kidneys to regulate volume and composition of urine.
    a) Prerenal causes: dehydration, hypovolemia
    b) Intrarenal causes: kidney infections, obstructions with damage, or nephrotoxic agents
    c) Postrenal obstruction
2. Glomerular filtration rate decreases, BUN and creatinine increase, output decreases, and sodium levels drop because of dilution of extracellular fluid.

B. Assessment
1. Meticulously measure intake and output.
2. Assess neurologic symptoms associated with the buildup of toxins and decrease of sodium (irritability, seizures).
3. Assess for signs of edema and congestive heart failure caused by the buildup of fluids.
4. Assess for metabolic acidosis and compensatory hyperventilation.
5. Be aware of kidney's role in stimulating erythropoiesis; assess for signs of anemia.

C. Intervention
1. Limit fluid intake depending on output; monitor IV lines to prevent fluid overload.
2. Correct electrolyte levels of sodium and potassium.
3. Assist child to eat concentrated foods without fluids; monitor protein and salt intake.
4. Prepare child for dialysis, if needed.
5. Promote good skin care; toxins are excreted through the skin, causing pruritus; keep nails trimmed and use a moisturizing cream.

IX. Hypospadias and epispadias

A. Introduction
1. Hypospadias is a congenital anomaly of the penis; the urethral opening may be anywhere along the ventral side of the penis.
2. Epispadias is an uncommon condition associated with exstrophy of the bladder; the urethral opening may be anywhere along the dorsal side of the penis.
3. Both conditions shorten the distance to the bladder, offering easier access to bacteria.

B. Assessment
1. Observe the angle of urination.
2. Assess the exit site.

C. Interventions
1. Keep the area clean to exclude bacteria.
2. Be aware that surgery involving implants or reconstruction may be needed to reduce the chance of UTIs and infertility.
3. Do not circumcise the infant with suspected hypospadias; the foreskin may be needed later during surgical repair.

X. Undescended testes

A. Introduction

1. The testes descend from the abdomen into the scrotum during the last 2 months of gestation.

2. If the testes are not descended at birth, they may descend on their own in a few weeks.

3. If the testes remain in the abdominal cavity after age 5, the seminiferous tubules may degenerate because of the increased body temperature in the abdomen, resulting in sterility.

B. Assessment

1. Palpate the scrotum (undescended testes are usually unilateral).

2. Visually inspect the scrotum; one side may appear underdeveloped.

C. Interventions

1. Expect diagnostic tests to check kidney function; the kidneys and the testes arise from the same germ tissue.

2. Be aware that surgery is usually performed between ages 2 and 5, with one suture passing through the testes and scrotum and attached to the thigh.

   a) Prevent pulling on the thigh suture postoperatively.

   b) The testes could reascend into the abdomen through the inguinal canal if the suture disconnects.

CHAPTER
12

Gastrointestinal Conditions

LEARNING OBJECTIVES

1. Describe acquired and congenital gastrointestinal problems that alter nutrition and hydration.

2. Assess and plan care for a child with vomiting and diarrhea.

3. Plan feeding interventions for a child with anomalies that interfere with ingesting nutrients.

4. Differentiate hepatitis A from hepatitis B.

I. Introduction

A. Many GI abnormalities originate during fetal life; they may or may not be detected during the neonatal period.

B. The signs and symptoms depend on which part of the GI tract is affected.

C. When obtaining a history for most GI conditions, it is important to obtain information on food habits (what is eaten, how it is prepared, how much is eaten, when does eating occur and with whom), vitamins and nutritional supplements that may be used, and normal bowel habits, including frequency, appearance, and the use of aids, such as laxatives or enemas.

D. Because of the processes of ingestion, digestion, absorption, and elimination, it is important to assess the timing of symptoms as they relate to eating and eliminating.

E. In assessing the abdomen, remember that auscultation must precede percussion and palpation to obtain an accurate assessment of bowel sounds.

F. While the newborn stomach expands from 20 ml at birth to as much as 90 ml by the end of the first week of life, the stomach holds up to 3,000 ml by late adolescence.

G. Remember that the infant's gut is immature during the first year of life; some products cannot be digested and are excreted in the stool, whereas other products may be absorbed more readily, possibly leading to the development of food allergy.

II. Vomiting

A. Introduction

1. Definition: the forceful emptying of stomach contents through the mouth—usually caused by a GI disorder (such as spasm of the duodenum, reverse peristalsis from blockage of the pylorus, reflux from an incompetent or lax esophageal sphincter, overdistention of the stomach from increased intake, or gastroenteritis), but may result from a non-GI disorder (such as increased intracranial pressure).

2. It is controlled by the medulla.

3. A "wet burp" or "spitting up" involves either dribbling of undigested liquids from the mouth and esophagus or their expulsion with the force of a burp and should be differentiated from vomiting.

B. Assessment
   1. Differentiate vomiting from a wet burp or spitting up.
   2. Review the child's history for frequency of episodes.
   3. Assess for accompanying symptoms, such as fever, nausea, headache, and diarrhea.
   4. Determine if the vomiting is projectile.
   5. Determine if the vomiting is related to intake or to other activities.
   6. Describe the vomitus: blood (hematemesis), bile, undigested or digested food, amount, force.
   7. Note presence or absence of nausea.
   8. Note the time since last ingestion of food.
   9. Assess abdomen: check for bowel sounds, note distention of abdomen or areas of pain.
      a) Measure abdomen with a paper tape at the widest point, usually the umbilicus; mark the point of measurement with a pen.
   10. Assess fluid and electrolyte balance, especially for dehydration (check skin turgor).
   11. Assess for metabolic alkalosis from the loss of stomach acids.
   12. Assess nutritional status, including growth and development.
   13. Evaluate feeding methods (amount of burping, air in nipple, feeding supine or sitting up).
C. Interventions
   1. Prevent aspiration by positioning the child on the side; maintain a patent airway; perform nasotracheal or bulb suctioning, if necessary.
   2. Withhold food and fluids to rest the stomach 4 to 6 hours; in severe vomiting, IV fluids may be needed.
   3. After a period of no vomiting and if an obstruction is not the cause, begin administering frequent small amounts of clear liquids.
      a) For infants: give Pedialyte.
      b) For older children: give flat noncarbonated ginger ale or cola.
   4. Administer antiemetic medications only to older children; they should not be used in infants; use the rectal or intramuscular route.
   5. Raise the head of the bed when feeding; place side-lying on right side or prone after feeding to prevent aspiration.

    6.   Provide skin and mouth care.

    7.   Measure intake and output as well as daily weight.

    8.   Monitor stool status.

III. Gastroesophageal reflux (GER)

A. Introduction

    1.   GER is the return of gastric contents into the esophagus from an incompetent or poorly developed esophageal sphincter.

    2.   The condition occurs almost immediately after eating and typically affects infants; it is also seen in premature infants and young children with spastic cerebral palsy and other conditions with decreased muscle tone.

    3.   Aspiration puts them at risk for pneumonia.

B. Assessment

    1.   Assess the relationship of vomiting to feedings, positioning, and the activity level immediately after feedings.

    2.   Assess for failure to thrive/poor weight gain.

    3.   Assess for aspiration of feedings; note any relationship between apnea and GER (many infants may be placed on apnea monitors).

    4.   Measure the pH of gastric contents.

C. Interventions

    1.   Administer medications 30 minutes before meals to maximize the benefits of the medications

        a)   Cimetidine (Tagamet), ranitidine (Zantac), and famotidine (Pepcid) are drugs used to reduce the amount of gastric acid present in gastric contents, thereby reducing esophagitis.

        b)   Metoclopramide (Reglan) decreases reflux by increasing pressure of the esophageal sphincter, increasing gastric emptying and increasing gastric peristalsis.

    2.   Provide thickened formula (1 tablespoon cereal/1 oz formula); will need to enlarge hole in nipple or use cross-cut nipple.

    3.   Feed child in an upright position.

    4.   Give small frequent feedings.

    5.   There is debate related to positioning after feeding. While prone with head of the bed raised for sleep has been recommended in the past, concern about SIDS now causes many to recommend the supine position for sleep.

    6.   Prepare for surgery (Nissen fundoplication) if necessary.

IV. Diarrhea

A. Introduction
1. Diarrhea is the increased frequency and amount and decreased consistency of stool.
2. It occurs when water in the bowel increases from osmotic pull, with electrolyte imbalance, or when peristalsis increases, preventing water from being absorbed.
3. It may accompany gastroenteritis, an inflammation of the lining of the stomach and intestines.
4. It can result from anatomic changes, malabsorption condition, GI allergies, or toxins.
5. It can lead to metabolic acidosis and dehydration.

B. Assessment
1. Note the amount, frequency, duration, consistency, appearance, and odor of stool; weigh diapers and note the amount of water loss.
2. Test stool for blood and other reducing substances, such as sugars, and for pH; obtain stool cultures, if ordered.
3. Assess for the presence of abdominal pain or cramping associated with stooling.
4. Assess the relationship between stooling and the time of eating or quality of intake.
5. Assess skin integrity around the anus.
6. Assess hydration status.
7. Assess abdomen; check bowel sounds, palpate for masses, distention, pain.

C. Interventions
1. For mild diarrhea, continue regular diet.
   a) Avoid fruit juices and soft drinks because of their high osmotic load.
2. For more serious diarrhea:
   a) For infants: Initiate unlimited amounts of Oral Rehydration Solutions (Pedialyte, Infalyte); continue breast feeding or formula.
   b) For children > than 1 year: Increase starchy foods in regular diet (rice cereal, oatmeal, toast, potatoes, carrots, white rice, applesauce, bananas); pretzels and salty crackers help meet sodium needs.
   c) IV fluids may be needed.
3. Use enteric precautions and good hand washing.
4. Measure intake and output.

5. Provide skin care around anus; apply a skin protectant; change diapers promptly.
6. Do not take child's temperature rectally.

V. Constipation

A. Introduction
1. Constipation is a decreased amount and increased consistency of stool compared to the patient's normal pattern (children do not need to have a daily bowel movement).
2. Constipation is not necessarily synonymous with straining.
3. It may be caused by diet low in liquids or high in fat and protein.

B. Assessment.
1. Note a hard, dry, infrequent stool.
2. Test stool for blood (guaiac test). Melena is dark, tarry stool usually associated with bleeding from the upper GI tract; it may be Hematest-positive from trauma to the rectal tissue from passing a hard mass; assess skin integrity around anus.
3. Ask child about abdominal pain during stooling or intermittent pain throughout the day.
4. Assess the child's diet for liquids, fiber, carbohydrates, and constipating foods.
5. Measure abdominal girth.
6. Note whether child is reluctant to use the toilet in school or is consciously retaining stool.

C. Interventions
1. Lubricate around the anus to ease the passage of hard stool (may have to remove stool digitally).
2. Administer stool softeners: suppositories, mineral oil, and docusate sodium (Colace).
3. Add corn syrup or liquid sugar preparations to the infant's formula to increase the osmotic load.
4. Add fiber or prune juice to the diet; increase fluid intake.
5. Administer enemas, if ordered; use isotonic solutions only.

VI. Cleft lip and palate

A. Introduction
1. Cleft lip and palate are a failure of the bone and tissue of the upper jaw and palate to fuse completely at the midline.

2. Cleft lip and palate are congenital defects, in some cases due to heredity but many other causes are implicated; the defect occurs in the 2nd and 3rd months of pregnancy.
3. The defects may be partial or complete, unilateral or bilateral, or may involve just the lip, just the palate, or both.
4. The condition requires a long-term team approach to address speech defects, dental and orthodontic problems, nasal defects, and possible alterations in hearing.
5. Because it results in facial disfigurement, the condition may cause shock, guilt, and grief for the parents and may interfere with parental bonding with the child.
6. Cleft lip and palate increase the risk of aspiration, because increased open space in the mouth causes some formula to exit through the nose with wet burps.
7. They also increase the risk of upper respiratory tract infection and otitis media, because the increased open space decreases natural defenses against bacterial invasion.

B. Assessment
1. Visually inspect and palpate the palate.
2. Assess the quality of the infant's suck; determine if the infant can form an airtight seal around a nipple.
3. Assess the child's ability to swallow.
4. Assess for abdominal distention from swallowed air.
5. Be alert for respiratory distress when feeding.

C. Interventions for cleft lip (preoperative)
1. Feed the infant slowly and in an upright position to decrease the risk of aspiration.
2. Burp often during feeding to eliminate swallowed air and decrease the risk of emesis.
3. Use a long soft lamb's nipple, a cleft palate nipple with a flap across the palate (palatal obturators), a medicine dropper, a syringe with rubber tubing attached to the end (aim nipple toward the side of the mouth), or manual compression to unite the edges of the cleft lip; all encourage sucking, promote oral muscle development, and enhance the infant's nutritional status.
4. Use gavage feedings if oral feedings are unsuccessful.
5. Administer a small amount of water after feedings to prevent formula from accumulating and becoming a medium for bacterial growth
6. Give small frequent feedings.

7. Hold infant while feeding and promote sucking between meals.
8. Provide psychological support to the parents; reinforce the likely success of surgery; point out the positive qualities of the infant
9. Tell parents that cleft lips are usually corrected when the infant is 10 weeks old and weighs 10 lb (4.5 kg); the infant must be free of respiratory infections at the time of surgery.

D. Interventions for postoperative cleft lip repair (cheiloplasty)
1. Be aware that cheiloplasty unites the lip and gum edges in anticipation of teeth eruption, provides a route for adequate nutrition and sucking, and improves the infant's appearance, which promotes parent-child bonding.
2. Maintain a patent airway; edema or narrowing of a previously large airway may make the infant appear to be in distress.
3. Observe for cyanosis, as the infant begins to breathe through the nose.
4. Maintain an intact suture line; keep the infant's hands away from the mouth by using restraints (protective devices), or pinning the sleeves to the shirt; Steri-Strips will be used to hold the suture line in place.
5. Prevent tension on the suture line by anticipating the infant's needs and preventing crying; do not place in prone position to avoid pressure on face (place in infant seat).
6. A mist tent may be ordered to keep the airway moist.
7. Give extra care and support, because the infant cannot meet emotional needs by sucking.
8. When feeding resumes, use a syringe with tubing to administer foods at the side of the mouth; this will prevent trauma to the suture line.
9. After feedings, place infant on right side to prevent aspiration.
10. To prevent crusts and scarring, clean suture line after each feeding by dabbing it with half-strength hydrogen peroxide or saline solution.
11. Monitor and treat for pain.

E. Interventions for cleft palate (preoperative)
1. Be aware that the infant must be weaned from the bottle or breast before cleft palate surgery; the infant must be able to drink from a cup.

2. Feed infant with a cleft palate nipple or a Teflon implant to enhance nutritional intake.
3. Surgery is usually scheduled at about 18 months of age (6-24 months) to allow for the growth of the palate and before the infant develops speech patterns; the infant must be free from ear and respiratory infections.
4. Teach the parents that the infant is susceptible to pathogens and otitis media from the altered position of the Eustachian tube.

F. Interventions for cleft palate (postoperative) (staphylorrhaphy)
1. Maintain a patent airway; position infant on the abdomen or side.
2. Anticipate edema and a decreased airway from palate closure; this may make the infant appear temporarily dyspneic.
3. Prevent trauma to the suture line by keeping hard or pointed objects (utensils, straws, frozen dessert sticks) away from the mouth; do not use suction catheters, except in emergency (use bulb syringe if necessary).
4. Use a cup to feed; do not use a nipple or pacifier.
5. Use elbow restraints to keep the child's hands out of the mouth.
6. Provide soft toys.
7. Start the child on clear liquids and progress to a soft diet; rinse the suture line by giving child a sip of water after each feeding.
8. Distract or hold child to try to keep the tongue away from the roof of the mouth.

VII. Esophageal atresia (EA) and tracheoesophageal fistula (TEF)

A. Introduction
1. An atresia is the termination of a passageway; it usually refers to a pathologic closure or the absence of a normal anatomic opening.
2. A fistula is a tubelike connection between two structures.
3. These conditions occur alone or in many combinations; they may be associated with other congenital defects, especially cardiac defects; TEF may be part of a syndrome called VACTERL (Vertebral defects, Anorectal malformations, Cardiac anomalies, TEF, EA, Renal defects, and Limb defects).

4. EA occurs when the proximal end of the esophagus ends in a blind pouch; food cannot enter the stomach via the esophagus.

5. TEF occurs when there is a connection between the esophagus and the trachea.

6. TEF may result in the reflux of gastric juice after feeding that can allow acidic stomach contents to cross the fistula, irritating the trachea.

7. EA with TEF occurs when either the distal end of the esophagus ends in a blind pouch and the proximal end of the esophagus is linked to the trachea via a fistula or when the proximal end of the esophagus ends in a blind pouch and the distal portion of the esophagus is connected to the trachea via a fistula; EA with TEF is the most common of these defects with EA alone being second most common.

8. Feed all newborns first with a few sips of sterile water to rule out these anomalies and to prevent the aspiration of formula into the lungs.

B. Assessment of TEF

1. Maternal history of polyhydramnios (excess amniotic fluid, since fetus is unable to swallow it).

2. Newborn may have excessive oral secretions.

3. Assess for choking, coughing, and intermittent cyanosis during feeding from food that goes through the fistula into the trachea; stop feeding if this occurs.

4. Observe for abdominal distention from air that goes through the fistula into the stomach.

5. Observe for tracheal irritation from gastric acids that reflux across the fistula.

C. Assessment of EA with TEF

1. Assess for all signs and symptoms of EA.

2. Observe for signs of respiratory distress: coughing, choking, and intermittent cyanosis.

D. Interventions

1. If EA or TEF is suspected, do not feed orally; a percutaneous endoscopic gastrostomy (PEG) tube may be inserted; keep the tube open and suspended above the child for release of gas.

2. Maintain a patent airway; have suction equipment available.

3. If feeding the child via gastrostomy tube after surgery, anticipate abdominal distention from air; keep the child upright during feedings to reduce the chance of regurgitated stomach contents and aspiration pneumonia, and keep the tube open and elevated before and after feedings.
4. Gastrostomy feeds should be administered only by gravity.
5. Explain to parents how the surgery ligates the TEF and reanastomoses the esophageal ends; expect a staged repair in many instances.

VIII. Pyloric stenosis

A. Introduction
   1. Pyloric stenosis is an increasing hyperplasia and hypertrophy of the circular muscle at the pylorus, which narrows the pyloric canal as it exits the stomach.
   2. The defect is most commonly seen in boys between age 2 weeks and 6 months.
   3. Emesis may be Hematest positive, but it will *not* contain bile; it will increase in amount and force as the obstruction increases and will become projectile.

B. Assessment
   1. Be aware that symptoms seldom appear during the first few weeks of life.
   2. May palpate for an olive-size bulge below the right costal margin.
   3. May observe for projectile emesis during or shortly after feedings (preceded by reverse peristaltic waves [going left to right] but not by nausea).
   4. Note that the child will resume eating after vomiting.
   5. Evaluate for poor weight gain and symptoms of malnutrition despite the child's apparent hunger.
   6. Assess for metabolic alkalosis and dehydration from frequent emesis.

C. Interventions
   1. Provide small, frequent, thickened feedings with the head of the bed elevated; burp the child frequently.
   2. Position the child to prevent the aspiration of vomitus, preferably on the right side.
   3. Correct an electrolyte imbalance.
   4. An NG tube may be inserted and kept open and elevated for gastric decompression.
   5. Prepare for pyloromyotomy.

IX. Intussusception

A. Introduction
   1. Intussusception is the telescoping or invagination of a bowel segment into itself, the most common site being the ileocecal valve; it usually occurs at about age 6 months.
   2. The condition may result from polyps, hyperactive peristalsis, an abnormal bowel lining, or for no known cause.
   3. Initially, it causes inflammation and swelling at the affected site; edema eventually causes obstruction and necrosis from occlusion of the blood supply to the bowel.
   4. Intussusception can be acute or chronic. Untreated, it may lead to peritonitis.

B. Assessment
   1. Note a sudden attack of acute abdominal pain in a previously well child; the child shrieks and draws the knees to the chest.
   2. Observe for an increase in bile-stained vomitus.
   3. Note the passage of a red currant jelly-like stool (red blood and mucus).
   4. Assess for a distended and tender abdomen.
   5. Note pallor and agitation.

C. Interventions
   1. Prepare for a barium enema or water-soluble contrast with air pressure to confirm the condition and reduce the invagination by hydrostatic pressure.
   2. Be aware that, if reduction of barium fails, surgery may be required to resect the gangrenous portion; a temporary colostomy may be necessary.

X. Congenital aganglionic megacolon/Hirschsprung's disease

A. Introduction
   1. Parasympathetic ganglionic cells are absent in a segment of the colon (usually at the distal end of the large intestines); the lack of nerve innervation causes a lack of or alteration in peristalsis in the affected part.
   2. As stool enters the affected part, it remains there until additional stool pushes it through; the affected part of the colon dilates; a mechanical obstruction may result.

B. Assessment
1. Observe the newborn for failure to pass meconium and stool.
2. Observe for liquid or ribbonlike stools; only fluid can pass the obstruction caused by stool.
3. Assess for a distended abdomen from stool impaction.
4. Assess for nausea, vomitus, anorexia, lethargy, weight loss, and failure to thrive.
5. Prepare for a biopsy of the large intestines to confirm condition.
6. Be alert for signs and symptoms of enterocolitis, volvulus, and shock, which can occur from this condition.

C. Interventions
1. Perform a digital exam to expand the anus enough to release impacted stool and provide temporary relief if the megacolon is near the rectum.
2. Do not treat liquid stool as diarrhea; it results from impaction.
3. Administer bowel irrigation with GoLYTELY via NG tube.
4. Administer isotonic enemas (saline solution or mineral oil) to evacuate the bowel; do not administer tap water because of the risk of water intoxication.
5. Be aware that total parenteral nutrition (TPN) may be used in place of oral feedings to rest the bowel.
6. Use low-residue diets and stool softeners to lessen stool bulk and thus decrease colonic irritation.
7. Be aware that surgery may be required to remove the aganglionic section.

XI. Imperforate anus

A. Introduction
1. An imperforate anus is an atresia of the anal opening; the infant may have no anal opening onto the skin wall, or the rectum may end in a blind pouch.
2. A fistula to the vagina in females or to the urethra in males may also be present.

B. Assessment
1. Observe to see from which orifice stool is excreted.
2. Assess for signs and symptoms of impaction from the inability to pass stool.
3. Measure abdominal girth to evaluate abdominal distention.

C. Interventions

1. Do not take the infant's temperature rectally unless stool has been excreted from the rectum.

2. After surgical reconstruction of the anus and the formation of a temporary colostomy, keep the infant prone with the hips elevated.

3. Keep site clean.

XII. Appendicitis

A. Introduction

1. Inflammation and obstruction of the blind sac at the end of the cecum results in ischemia, gangrene, perforation, and peritonitis.

2. Suggested causes include infections, dietary intake, constipation, and parasites.

3. It is common in school-age children.

B. Assessment

1. Symptoms are variable, making a quick and accurate diagnosis difficult.

2. Assess for abdominal pain and tenderness that begins as diffuse, then localizes in the lower right quadrant at McBurney point.

3. Note fever, an increased white blood cell count, and behavioral changes.

4. Note rebound tenderness, especially in the lower right quadrant (more pain occurs when the hand is released than when the hand presses down on the abdomen).

5. Assess for decreased bowel sounds, nausea, vomiting, and anorexia.

6. Assess for abdominal distention, abdominal rigidity, and guarding.

7. Note symptoms of peritonitis if a rupture occurs (fever, sudden relief of pain followed by a diffuse pain).

C. Interventions

1. Position the child preoperatively in a semi-Fowler or right side–lying position.

2. Child may return from surgery with a drain and an NG tube attached to low intermittent suction.

3. Resume oral nutrition when bowel sounds reappear.

4. Administer antibiotics and pain medications.

5. Prepare for surgery, if indicated.

XIII. Inflammatory bowel disease

A. Introduction

1. Inflammatory bowel disease consists of Crohn's disease (regional enteritis) and ulcerative colitis.

   a) Ulcerative colitis involves symmetrical and contiguous GI ulcers; Crohn's disease involves asymmetrical and patchy lesions.

   b) Ulcerative colitis causes more blood loss than Crohn's disease.

   c) Ulcerative colitis attacks the mucosa of the bowel; Crohn's disease affects all layers of the bowel wall.

   d) Crohn's disease involves enlarged regional lymph nodes.

   e) Ulcerative colitis usually involves the large intestines; Crohn's disease can occur at any point along the GI tract.

2. Inflammatory bowel disease is diagnosed on the basis of results of a barium enema, biopsy of the GI mucosa, and stool studies.

3. Edema and inflammation of the bowel produces ulceration, bleeding, diarrhea, and abdominal distention.

4. Chronic exacerbations may delay growth and development, including sexual development.

5. The disease, which commonly occurs in adolescents, is exacerbated by emotional factors, but its cause is unknown.

B. Assessment

1. Assess for weight loss, anorexia, nausea, and vomiting.

2. Test stool for blood.

3. Observe for diarrhea.

4. Test for anemia and signs of hypovolemia.

5. Assess for arthritis.

C. Interventions

1. Administer analgesics and antispasmodics to decrease abdominal pain.

2. Administer corticosteroids to decrease bowel inflammation.

3. Administer immunomodulators (methotrexate and cyclosporine).

4. Promote stress reduction through relaxation, distraction, and enhanced self-image and self-esteem.

5. Withhold food and fluids, using parenteral nutrition in place of feeding to rest the bowel; or provide a high-protein, high-calorie, low-residue, low-fat diet with vitamin supplementation.

6. Be aware that when conditions are not amenable to medical treatment, a colectomy, ileostomy, or ileo-anal pull-through may be performed.

XIV. Celiac disease

A. Introduction
1. An absence of an enzyme in the intestinal mucosal cells causes the villi of the proximal small intestine to atrophy and decreases intestinal absorption.
2. The disease is a response to gluten intolerance (inability to absorb rye, oat, wheat, and barley glutens).
3. Related to IgA deficiency and the early introduction of protein solids, celiac disease usually occurs 2 to 4 months after solid foods are introduced.

B. Assessment
1. Assess for steatorrhea (fatty stools) and chronic diarrhea from fat malabsorption.
2. Assess for generalized malnutrition and failure to thrive from the malabsorption of protein and carbohydrates.
3. Evaluate for osteoporosis and coagulation difficulty from the malabsorption of fat-soluble vitamins.
4. Assess for abdominal pain from calcium depletion.
5. Observe for irritability from anemia.
6. Prepare the child for an intestinal biopsy to diagnose the condition.

C. Interventions
1. Eliminate gluten from the diet.
2. Give child corn and rice products, soy and potato flour, Probana formula, and all fresh fruits.
3. Replace vitamins and calories; give small frequent meals.
4. Attempt to prevent the disease by delaying the introduction of solid foods until after age 6 months.

XV. Necrotizing enterocolitis

A. Introduction
1. Necrotizing enterocolitis is common in premature infants during the neonatal period.
2. It can result from various factors that cause vascular compromise, such as asphyxia.
3. Blood flow to the GI tract is compromised as oxygenated blood is diverted to the brain and heart.
4. Bowel mucosa becomes necrotic, thereby decreasing protective mucus.
5. Gas-forming bacteria invade the necrotic tissue.
6. Formula feedings may exacerbate conditions, because food provides a nutritional base for bacteria to grow.

B. Assessment
1. Observe for abdominal distention.
2. Monitor for an increase in gastric residual (the amount not digested and left in the stomach from the previous feeding); note vomiting.
3. Assess stool for blood and sugar.
4. Note lethargy, apnea with bradycardia, hypotension, and an unstable temperature.
5. Check abdominal X-ray for increased GI gas.
6. Note an increase in daily abdominal girth measurements.

C. Interventions
1. Rest the bowel; use parenteral nutrition and allow nothing by mouth.
2. Use an NG tube connected to low suction to decompress the abdomen
3. Administer antibiotics as prescribed.
4. Reduce stress by maintaining body temperature and by handling the infant only when necessary.
5. Prepare family for the possibility of a colostomy if the necrotic bowel is surgically removed; this may result in short-bowel syndrome resulting in possible lifelong reliance on TPN.
6. Be aware that abdominal perforation can lead to overwhelming sepsis, shock, and death.

XVI. Biliary atresia

A. Introduction
1. Biliary atresia is the obliteration or absence of extrahepatic biliary structures; its cause is unknown.
2. This congenital anomaly can cause liver failure and death.

B. Assessment
1. Observe for jaundice early in infancy.
2. Observe for dark urine from hyperbilirubinemia and pale stools from the absence of bile.
3. Assess for hepatomegaly, ascites, and splenomegaly.
4. Expect irritability.
5. Assess for failure to thrive or poor weight gain from decreased absorption of fat-soluble vitamins.
6. Note whether laboratory tests show increased conjugated bilirubin, cholesterol, alkaline phosphatase levels, and prolonged prothrombin time.
7. Prepare for a liver biopsy to diagnose the condition.

C. Interventions
1. Give fat-soluble vitamins in water-miscible form.
2. Be aware that, if no treatable condition is identified, surgery (the Kasai procedure) can be done to form a substitute duct, but this is not a permanent correction.
3. Be aware that a liver transplantation may be done for uncorrectable atresia.

XVII. Parasitic worms

A. Introduction
1. Worms are acquired through the skin or by ingesting dirt or raw vegetables containing helminth eggs.
2. The eggs hatch and travel by the GI tract or blood to the gut, where they attach and thrive.
3. Infestation is commonly caused by unsanitary disposal of stool and lack of hand washing.
4. Symptoms depend on the worm type and load, as well as on the degree of intestinal damage and irritation.
5. Pinworm is the most common worm infestation.
    a) The worms are 5 to 10 mm long.
    b) They live in the cecum and crawl to the anus at night to deposit eggs in the perianal area.
    c) The cycle repeats itself when the child scratches the anus and puts the hand to the mouth.
    d) The condition can be diagnosed by using an adhesive tape test.
        (1) Tape is put across the anus at night.
        (2) The worms lay eggs on the tape.
        (3) The tape can be removed in the morning and used as a microscope slide to diagnose.
    e) Oral medications for pinworms will color the stool red; this is not related to bleeding.

B. Assessment
1. Assess for bloody diarrhea leading to anemia; test for blood in stool.
2. Assess for failure to thrive related to malabsorption.
3. Assess for abdominal distention, anorexia, nausea, and vomiting.
4. Expect intense anal pruritus and scratching if the child is infested with pinworms.

C. Interventions
1. Teach the child and parents sanitary stool disposal techniques.
2. Review proper hand washing before meals and after toileting.
3. Urge them to wash fruits and vegetables before eating.
4. Advise the child to wear shoes in infested areas.
5. Administer medication appropriate to the type of infestation.

XVIII. Viral hepatitis

A. Introduction
1. Inflammation of the liver due to one of five or more viruses
   a) Hepatitis A virus is passed by the fecal-oral route, most commonly by poor sanitation or in day care centers; incubation period is 4 weeks, and GI symptoms are usually mild. Good hand washing after toileting and diaper changes, as well as environmental controls, can prevent this form.
   b) Hepatitis B virus is transmitted via blood and body secretions, as well as vertically from mother to fetus; it can be acute or chronic and can result in the long-term sequelae of cirrhosis, liver cancer, or fulminant hepatitis; incubation is 50 to 180 days.
   c) Hepatitis C virus is predominantly parenterally spread with an incubation of 14 to 180 days; it causes severe liver damage and frequently results in the need for a liver transplant.
   d) Hepatitis D virus occurs in conjunction with hepatitis B virus.
   e) Hepatitis E virus is similar in transmission to hepatitis A.
2. Diagnosis is made by identifying the antigenic markers and the body's immune response.

B. Assessment
1. Prodromal symptoms may include anorexia, malaise, easily fatigued, and possibly a fever.
2. Assess for nausea, vomiting, epigastric or right upper quadrant abdominal discomfort.
3. Assess for hepatomegaly and increased abdominal girth.
4. Assess for jaundice, dark urine, and pale stools.
5. Assess liver function tests (transaminases) and bilirubin levels.

6.   Assess for a history of blood transfusions, sexual activity, needle sharing of any substances, poor sanitation, ingestion of hepatotoxic drugs, exposure to blood or body secretions of an infected individual, as in diaper changing.

C.   Interventions
1.   Administer hepatitis immune globulin (HBIG) for contact with hepatitis B.
2.   Administer hepatitis immunization series to infants and adolescents if not already protected.
3.   Implement standard precautions; stress good hand washing and hygienic environmental measures.
4.   Management for noncritical cases is supportive and symptomatic and usually takes place in the home environment; promote rest, fluids, and good nutrition.

XIV.   The child receiving enteral feedings

A.   These include feedings delivered directly into the stomach or intestines by either an NG tube, a nasojejunal tube, or a gastrostomy tube.
1.   NG tubes stiffen when left in place for long periods of time and can cause irritation to mucous membranes.
2.   Soft NG tubes are made of Silastic and come with a wire stylet that is used only for inserting the tube and then is removed.
3.   When inserting an enteral tube, if resistance is encountered, withdraw the tube and try again; use of force may cause perforation.
    a)   pH testing of aspirate is the most reliable way to verify placement, secondary to X-ray.
4.   Gastrostomy tubes are placed surgically or by endoscopic methods (PEG tube); a gastrostomy tube that is skin level is called a "button" gastrostomy.

B.   Feedings can be continuous or intermittent; they can be delivered by a pump or by gravity.

C.   Nonnutritive sucking has multiple benefits for the infant receiving enteral feeds, including improved weight gain, increased alert states, and decreased restlessness.

XX. Acetaminophen poisoning

A. Introduction
   1. Acetaminophen is an analgesic, antipyretic agent that does not inhibit platelet aggregation and does not affect inflammation as does aspirin.
   2. Hepatotoxicity occurs at plasma levels greater than 200 µg/ml.

B. Assessment
   1. Assess for GI distress, such as nausea, vomiting, diarrhea, and abdominal pain.
   2. Monitor for liver damage 24 to 36 hours after the overdose.

C. Intervention
   1. Administer an antidote, such as acetylcysteine (Mucomyst).

CHAPTER
13

Endocrine/Metabolic Conditions

LEARNING OBJECTIVES

1. Assess and plan care for the child with type 1 diabetes.

2. Describe conditions resulting from hyposecretion of the pituitary gland.

3. Assess alterations in growth and development from the hyposecretion of thyroid hormones.

I. Introduction

A. Endocrine glands (pituitary, thyroid, parathyroids, adrenal, pancreas, ovaries, testes) are ductless and secrete hormones directly into the circulation.

B. The hormones are transported throughout the body and affect metabolic processes and functions.

C. Hormone production and secretion are regulated through a negative feedback loop that interrelates many of the endocrine glands.

D. Endocrine dysfunction may result from hyposecretion or hypersecretion of hormones.

E. The endocrine system is responsible for regulating growth, metabolism, fluid and electrolyte balance, sexual reproduction, and the body's response to stress.

F. The gonads produce hormones responsible for pubertal changes.

G. The pituitary gland releases growth hormone.
1. It is called the master gland because it controls the release of other hormones.
2. The anterior lobe affects growth (growth hormone), sexual development (follicle-stimulating hormone, luteinizing hormone, prolactin), thyroid (thyroid-stimulating hormone), adrenal function (adrenocorticotropic hormone [ACTH]), and skin pigment (melanocyte-stimulating hormone).
3. The posterior lobe influences uterine contractions (oxytocin) and produces antidiuretic hormone (vasopressin, which has its effect on the kidneys).
   a) Syndrome of inappropriate antidiuretic hormone (SIADH) may be due to brain tumor, head trauma or surgery, or brain infection.
   b) SIADH causes an increased release of antidiuretic hormone (ADH) that tells the kidneys to reabsorb too much water; this results in decreased output, expanded fluid volume in the vessels, and diluted sodium concentration (hyponatremia).

H. The thyroid secretes T_3, T_4 (thyroxine), and calcitonin.

I. The adrenal cortex secretes mineralocorticoids (aldosterone), sex hormones (estrogen, progesterone, and androgens), and glucocorticoids (cortisol and corticosterone); the adrenal medulla secretes epinephrine (adrenaline) and norepinephrine.

J.   The ovaries also secrete estrogen and progesterone; the testes secrete testosterone.

K.   The endocrine portion of the pancreas secretes insulin (beta cells) and glucagon (alpha cells).

L.   Insulin production and ADH release are not under pituitary control.

II. Deficient anterior pituitary hormone: Pituitary dwarfism

A.   Introduction
   1.   Hypopituitarism results in decreased growth hormone.
   2.   The cause can be idiopathic or from brain tumor, trauma, or lesions.
   3.   Decreased pituitary function can decrease the release of precursors for thyroid, adrenal, and gonadotropin functions.

B.   Assessment
   1.   Review the child's history for normal birth length; then assess for a gradual decrease in height compared with peers.
   2.   Observe for short stature but normal body proportions.
   3.   Note that, physically, the child appears younger than expected; the child is usually well nourished.
   4.   Note that bone age studies reveal growth retardation.
   5.   Note that mental age approximates chronologic age; the child has normal intelligence.
   6.   Assess for delayed but normal pubertal development.
   7.   Assess the teeth; dental anomalies may occur when permanent teeth erupt because of growth retardation of the jaw.
   8.   Review the family's history to rule out a genetic reason for the lag in height.

C.   Interventions
   1.   Administer growth hormone to help the child catch up physically to peers.
   2.   Treat the child according to mental age, not bone age or height.
   3.   Provide social and psychological support to help the child cope.

III. Hypersecretion of anterior pituitary hormone: Gigantism or acromegaly

A.   Overview
   1.   May be from hyperplasia of the pituitary cells or a pituitary tumor

2. May present different symptoms depending on whether hypersecretion of growth hormone occurs before or after the epiphyseal plates close

B. Assessment
   1. Note that bone age studies are normal.
   2. Assess for signs and symptoms of gigantism if the increased release of growth hormone occurs before the closure of the epiphyseal plates.
      a) Elongation and enlargement of the long bones, facial bones, and accompanying body tissue
      b) Late closure of the fontanels
      c) Proportional body growth
   3. Assess for signs and symptoms of acromegaly if the increased release of growth hormone occurs after the closure of the epiphyseal plates.
      a) Enlargement of the hands, feet, nose, tongue, and jaw
      b) Thickening of the skin and coarseness of facial features

C. Interventions
   1. Be aware that radiation may be used to retard growth.
   2. Provide social and emotional support to help the child (especially the female) deal with large size.

IV. Hyposecretion of thyroid gland hormone

A. Overview
   1. The thyroid regulates the basal metabolic rate.
   2. The decreased secretion of thyroid hormones results from the decreased development of the thyroid gland or from medications that suppress hormone production; the thyroid depends on dietary iodine and tyrosine to function normally.

B. Assessment
   1. For congenital hypothyroidism, evaluate for mental retardation that develops as the disorder progresses if treatment is not initiated.
   2. Observe for short stature with the persistence of infant proportions
      a) Legs shorter in relation to trunk size
      b) Short thick neck
   3. Observe for an enlarged tongue.
   4. Assess for hypotonia.

5. Assess for delayed dentition.
6. For acquired hypothyroidism, assess for signs and symptoms of slow basal metabolic rate.
    a) Easy weight gain
    b) Cool body and skin temperature
    c) Slow pulse
    d) Dry, scaly skin
    e) Decreased perspiration
    f) Constipation
    g) Fatigue and tiredness
    h) Mental sluggishness
7. Assess for goiter.
8. Note that blood tests show low serum T_3 and T_4 levels.

D. Interventions
1. Administer oral thyroid hormone (thyroxine).
2. Administer supplemental vitamin D to prevent rickets resulting from rapid bone growth.
3. Monitor growth and development.

V. Hyperfunction of the adrenal gland: Cushing syndrome

A. Overview
1. Also called hyperadrenocorticism
2. High cortisol levels produced, resulting in the decreased secretion of ACTH
3. Often due to a tumor in the pituitary gland
4. Can also be due to prolonged or excessive use of corticosteroids for other conditions

B. Assessment
1. Central obesity: increased accumulation of fat on chest, upper back, and face (moon face); weigh daily.
2. Increased gluconeogenesis; decreased glucose tolerance; test sugar levels.
3. Increased protein catabolism leads to muscle weakness/atrophy.
4. Assess skin daily for purplish striae on skin; easy bruising.
5. Be aware of possibility of osteoporosis with susceptibility to bone fractures.
6. Assess for acne.
7. Assess for facial hair growth/hirsutism.
8. Assess for decreased linear growth, as ACTH inhibits the action of growth hormone.

9. Assess BP for hypertension.
10. Assess for mood disorders.
11. Assess for poor wound healing.

C. Interventions
   1. Prepare for surgery, if needed to remove a tumor.
   2. Work with medical staff to slowly taper exogenous corticosteroids, depending on the condition for which they are given.
   3. Promote a clean environment because of decreased immunity to infection.
   4. If steroids are needed, administer them early in the morning and on an alternate-day basis, if possible.
   5. Anorexia and nausea may be relieved by nasogastric decompression.
   6. Be supportive related to the child's mood changes, as these may not improve for months.

VI. Type 1 diabetes mellitus (DM)

A. Overview
   1. It is the most common cause of diabetes in children (previously called juvenile diabetes).
   2. It is a chronic systemic disorder most commonly diagnosed between ages 10 and 14 but can occur at any age from infancy to age 30.
   3. Predisposition to the disease may be genetically passed by human leukocyte antigen in 20% of cases.
   4. An autoimmune attack occurs against the beta cells of the pancreas approximately 1 week after an immune insult, such as an upper respiratory tract infection, although autoantibodies may be present up to 9 years before onset of clinical symptoms.
      a) No insulin is produced, and the cells cannot use glucose; excess glucose in the blood spills into the urine.
      b) The increased blood glucose can act as an osmotic diuretic, resulting in dehydration, hypotension, and renal shutdown.
      c) Without glucose, the cells are starving (resulting in signals of hunger and increased food intake [polyphagia]).
      d) The body attempts to compensate for lost energy by converting triglycerides to fatty acids, which then form ketones with resulting metabolic acidosis.

5. Two random plasma glucose levels of >126 mg/dl in someone who is asymptomatic or two random plasma glucose levels >200 mg/dl in someone who is asymptomatic or one high plasma glucose level in someone with symptoms is grounds for a diagnosis of DM.
6. Children test a minimum of 4 times per day.
7. The child appears thin and possibly malnourished.
8. The child is insulin dependent.
   a) Hyperglycemia can result from increased intake of sugar, decreased use of insulin, decreased exercise with no decrease in food intake, increased stressors, infection, or cortisone use.
   b) Hypoglycemia (insulin shock) can result from increased insulin use, excessive exercise, or failure to eat.
9. If it cannot be determined whether a stuporous diabetic is suffering from hypoglycemia or hyperglycemia, treat for hypoglycemia.

B. Assessment for hyperglycemia
   1. Ask about polyuria (frequent urination), polydipsia (thirst), and polyphagia (hunger); these are cardinal signs and symptoms.
   2. Note weakness, fatigue, headache, nausea, vomiting, and abdominal cramps.
   3. Test blood sugar; >240 mg/dl is hyperglycemia.
   4. Test for glycosuria (when glucose reaches 200 mg/dl, renal tubules cannot absorb all of the sugar, causing it to spill into the urine) and ketonuria using dipstick, Clinitest, Acetest, Keto-Diastix, or Tes-Tape.
      a) Note hyperglycemia as measured by finger stick or blood glucose test.
   5. Observe for dry, flushed skin.
   6. Note "fruity" breath odor.
   7. Long-term control of blood sugar is monitored by the glycosylated hemoglobin A_{1c} (HgbA$_{1c}$); hemoglobin in RBCs attaches to sugar; RBCs live for 90 to 120 days; HgbA$_{1c}$ measures the average amount of blood sugar over the past 90 to 120 days. A HgbA$_{1c}$ of 7 is the goal.

C. Interventions for hyperglycemia
   1. Administer rapid-acting or regular insulin for fast action.
   2. Give fluids without sugar to flush out acetone.
   3. Follow treatment for acidosis.
   4. Monitor blood sugar.

D. Assessment for hypoglycemia
    1. Blood sugar tests <70 mg/dl.
    2. Note time when insulin was administered and if it is the peak time of its action (regular insulin peaks 2-4 hours after administration; intermediate insulin peaks 4-12 hours after administration).
    3. Has child eaten or exercised?
    4. Assess for increased vital signs.
    5. Observe for sweating.
    6. Note tremors.
    7. Observe for behavior changes (slow thinking, confusion, irritability, poor coordination).

E. Interventions for hypoglycemia
    1. Give a fast-acting carbohydrate, such as a small tube of gel form cake icing, 4 oz orange juice, or ½ cup regular soda pop, followed later by a protein source.
    2. Follow seizure precautions.

F. Insulins
    1. Lispro/Humalog (clear, rapid acting): onset 10 to 15 minutes, peaks in 30 to 90 minutes.
    2. Regular (clear, fast acting): onset 30 minutes, peaks in 2 to 3 hours.
    3. NPH /Lente (cloudy, intermediate acting): onset 2 to 4 hours, peaks in 6 to 12 hours; Lente is now replaced by Lantus, a clear, long-acting insulin that is used only for basal needs, with no peaks, and it is not related to meals (do not mix Lantus with other insulins).
    4. Administration
        a) When giving both types, draw up clear insulin first to prevent contamination (remember, Lantus *cannot* be mixed with other insulins).
        b) To prevent air bubbles, do not shake the vial; intermediate forms are suspensions and should be gently rotated.
        c) Rotate injection sites to prevent lipodystrophy.
        d) Make sure the child eats when the insulin peaks.
        e) Insulin requirement may be altered with illness, stress, growth, food intake, and exercise; blood glucose measurements are the best way to determine insulin adjustment.
        f) Insulin may be given by syringe and needle, an insulin pen, or an insulin pump.

    5. Insulin is administered twice a day, at a minimum (before breakfast and dinner); administration may be more frequent.

    6. Dosage is based on either amount of carbohydrates consumed or blood sugar.

    7. Store unopened vials in refrigerator; open vials may be stored at room temperature and are good for 1 month; insulin pens are good for 14 to 30 days, depending on the type of insulin.

G. Meal planning

    1. May require a prescribed number of carbohydrates (one carbohydrate choice is 15 g carbohydrate) or an exchange list for carbohydrates

H. Complications of diabetes

    1. Life expectancy is shortened by one third.

    2. Nephropathy is the primary cause of death.

    3. Premature atherosclerosis with vascular insufficiency (leading to heart disease and stroke) and renal failure are possible.

    4. Retinopathy may lead to blindness.

    5. Poor wound healing is characteristic.

    6. Predisposition to infection is characteristic.

I. Honeymoon period

    1. This is a one-time remission of the symptoms, which occurs shortly after insulin treatment is started.

    2. It is a final effort by the pancreas to produce insulin

    3. The child can be insulin free for up to 1 year but may need oral hypoglycemics.

    4. Symptoms of hyperglycemia will reappear, and the child will be insulin dependent for life.

VII. Type 2 DM

A. Overview

    1. Typically seen in obese and overweight children who are physically inactive

    2. Increasing in epidemic proportions; 30% to 45% of DM in children is type 2

    3. Caused by both genetic and environmental factors; 50% to 80% have a parent with a family history of diabetes

    4. Will be the biggest cause of morbidity and early mortality for the next generation of adults

    5. Occurs as a result of insulin resistance plus some insulin deficiency; insulin resistance results in diminished liver, muscle, and adipose tissue sensitivity to insulin

B. Assessment
1. Assess for acanthosis nigricans, a thickening and hyperpigmentation of the skin at the neck and flexural areas.
2. Assess for hypertension, hyperlipidemia.
3. Assess for sleep apnea.

C. Interventions
1. Intervention includes a combination of exercise, weight loss, and medication (if needed).
2. Metformin (Glucophage) decreases glucose production by the liver.

VIII. Inborn errors of metabolism

A. Overview
1. These include multiple conditions resulting from altered biochemistry; enzyme abnormalities resulting in accumulation of a reactant that may or may not have toxic effects; most are autosomal recessive.
2. Phenylketonuria (PKU) results from a defect in hydroxylation of phenylalanine to form tyrosine; the resulting buildup of dietary phenylalanine results in brain damage and mental retardation. The urine has a musty odor.
3. Galactosemia is a deficiency in a galactose enzyme that results in liver failure, renal tubular problems, and cataracts.
4. Maple syrup urine disease (MSUD) is a deficiency of the decarboxylase that degrades some amino acids resulting in altered tonicity and seizures; the urine has the odor of maple syrup.

B. Assessment
1. Test urine and blood samples after the first 24 hours of feedings.
2. For neonates discharged before 24 hours of birth, ensure that during home visits the nurse obtains blood samples for testing and obtains rapid test results; refer for abnormal test results.

C. Interventions
1. For PKU, eliminate dietary phenyl ketones, such as in high-protein foods (milk, meat, eggs, beans, and nuts).
2. For galactosemia, eliminate dietary galactose (generally available as lactose).
3. For MSUD, restrict branched-chain amino acids in the diet, as in high-protein foods.

CHAPTER
14

Central Nervous System Conditions

LEARNING OBJECTIVES

1. Describe alterations in sensory, integrative, and motor functions of the central nervous system.

2. Discuss interventions to promote the growth, development, safety, and comfort of a child with alterations in any component of the sensory motor arc.

3. Differentiate among the multiple disorders that can increase intracranial pressure.

I. Chapter overview

Knowledge of normal central nervous system function provides a foundation for understanding conditions associated with its altered functioning. Rapid assessment and prompt intervention are necessary to stabilize the patient, promote optimal level of functioning, and prevent complications. Monitoring for signs and symptoms of increased intracranial pressure is crucial.

II. Introduction

A. Central nervous system (CNS) functions
   1. The CNS is a communication system that receives sensory stimuli from the external (exteroceptors) or internal (interoceptors or proprioceptors) environment.
      a) It perceives, integrates, interprets, or retains the stimulus in memory.
      b) The stimulus commonly results in a motor response.
   2. The five senses are vision, hearing, touch, taste, and smell.
   3. The infant's early responses are primarily reflexive; the infant learns to discriminate stimuli and bring motor responses under conscious control.
   4. Language helps the older child improve and increase perception.

B. CNS disorders
   1. Defects in any phase of the CNS can alter sensory, integrative, or motor function; the degree of disability depends on the amount and location of damage.
   2. The damaged nerve cells cannot be replaced.
   3. The later a part of the nervous system develops in embryonic life, the more susceptible it is to injury.
   4. Overload or deprivation of stimuli results in altered CNS functioning.
   5. Flaccid muscles usually indicate a CNS disorder.

III. Impaired vision

A. Blindness
   1. Introduction
      a) Vision provides a spatial sense and has a symbolic value.
      b) The newborn fixates on light; binocular vision develops at age 4 months; vision matures at age 6.
      c) The blind child has no visual memories; the child cannot see perspective or reflection and is less motivated to explore.

2. Assessment of vision
    a) Observe the child face to face.
        (1) The child's eyes should be at the same level.
        (2) The juncture of the pinna will form a straight line from the lateral corner of the eye.
    b) Assess visual acuity using the Snellen or Lea symbol chart (ages 3 to 6) or the Snellen letter chart (over 6) or the Titmus machine.
    c) Check for strabismus.
    d) Check for nystagmus.
3. Assessment for altered vision
    a) Evaluate the child's growth and developmental status.
        (1) The child may be slow in acquiring behavior patterns.
        (2) The child may appear delayed in posture control and in acquiring developmental tasks.
    b) Observe the child's behavior.
        (1) The child may be at a disadvantage in unfamiliar surroundings.
        (2) The child may be temporarily more dependent than usual.
        (3) The child may have frightening and intimidating experiences (such as the feeling of falling) that inhibit exploration.
        (4) The child may engage in self-stimulating behaviors, such as eye rubbing or body rocking.
    c) Assess the child's ability to fixate on objects, follow a moving light, or reach out to objects.
    d) Note whether the child initiates eye contact with the parents.
    e) Observe for a head tilt or frequent blinking or squinting.
    f) Ask the parents if the child holds the head very close to books or other objects.
    g) Ask the parents if the child walks or crawls into furniture or people.
4. Interventions
    a) Assist the child in learning to understand the world through the other senses.
    b) Encourage the parents to treat the child normally and to stimulate the child's other senses via play and touch.

  c) Encourage exploration and independence; arrange furniture to promote mobility and safety.

  d) Act as the child's safety advocate.

  e) Announce yourself on entering the room and explain intended actions before doing them.

  f) Explain strange sounds to the child.

  g) Teach the parents tips for the child with partial sight; seat the child at front of the classroom, use large-print materials, and use contrasting wall colors.

B. Amblyopia (lazy eye)

 1. Introduction

  a) Amblyopia can result from strabismus.

  b) It can cause vision loss through disuse.

 2. Assessment

  a) Note decreased visual acuity in the affected eye despite optical correction.

  b) Assess for central vision loss in the suppressed eye.

 3. Interventions

  a) Patch the healthy eye.

  b) For best results, refer the child for treatment before age 6.

C. Conjunctivitis (pinkeye)

 1. Introduction

  a) Conjunctivitis is an infection of the conjunctiva caused by bacteria, virus, fungus, or allergy.

  b) An infection not caused by allergy can be highly contagious; may return to school after being on antibiotics 24 hours (for bacterial conjunctivitis).

 2. Assessment

  a) Note if the child complains of itching, burning, or scratchiness beneath the eyelid.

  b) Note photophobia, edema of the eyelids, and reddened conjunctiva.

  c) Assess for discharge from the eye.

 3. Interventions

  a) Follow infection control measures carefully; wash hands thoroughly; use asepsis when handling eye secretions because of the high risk for possible infection transmission.

  b) Do not let the child share pillows, towels, or bed linens with others.

  c) Administer ophthalmic medications; apply ointment from the inner to the outer canthus.

IV. Impaired hearing

A. Introduction
   1. The ability to hear influences communication, speech, and intellectual functioning.
   2. The infant should turn the head to locate a sound; hearing is fully developed at birth.
   3. Hearing loss is conductive (middle ear), sensorineural (inner ear or eighth cranial nerve), or both; it can be caused by infection, inflammation, pressure, heredity, or noise.
   4. Cerumen accumulation decreases auditory acuity.
   5. Alterations in the location or shape of the ears warrant an evaluation of kidney function, because these organs develop simultaneously in utero.

B. Assessment
   1. Note if the child does not react to or turn to locate a sound or does not respond to being repeatedly called by name unless the speaker's lips are visible.
   2. Note if the child does not respond to simple verbal commands or questions or is not soothed by music or by being read to.
   3. Assess speech development.
      a) The child with impaired hearing does not develop recognizable speech.
      b) The child fails to vocalize, remains at the babbling stage, or shows decreased babbling.
   4. Review the child's history for poor academic performance, tendency to listen to television and radio at high volumes, straining to hear, or speech difficulty, which may indicate mild hearing loss.
   5. Assess for a history of premature birth, meningitis, or use of ototoxic medication, for example, gentamicin; assess for maternal prenatal history of rubella.

C. Interventions
   1. Promote communication via sign language or verbal communication.
   2. Encourage face-to-face communication to develop lipreading.
   3. Speak clearly and distinctly, but do not exaggerate the pronunciation of words; do not shout; interact in a well-lit environment.
   4. Wait for the child's attention before speaking.

5. Decrease additional noise in the room.
6. Allow only one person to speak at a time.
7. Use multisensory approaches to develop speech; have the child touch your lips and feel the vibrations of vocal cords.
8. Promote peer interaction.
9. Use demonstration to explain procedures and treatments before initiating them.
10. Be aware that conductive hearing loss may be remedied by a hearing aid.

V. Mental retardation/cognitive impairment

A. Introduction
   1. According to the American Association on Mental Retardation, mental retardation is a disability that involves significant limitations both in intellectual functioning and in adaptive behavior as expressed in conceptual, social, and practical adaptive skills and is manifested during the developmental period (prior to age 18).
   2. IQ alone is not the only criterion for mental retardation; individuals who adapt well to the environment may not necessarily be considered mentally retarded.
   3. Degrees of mental retardation are as follows:
      a) Mild (IQ 50-55 to 70): 80% of those classified as mentally retarded
         (1) Educable to a mental age of 8 to 12
         (2) Capable of most independent activities of daily living
      b) Moderate (IQ 35-40 to 50-55): 15% of those classified as mentally retarded
         (1) Includes most of those with Down syndrome
         (2) Can be trained in self-care to the mental age of 3 to 7
      c) Severe (IQ 20-25 to 35-40)
         (1) Achieves the mental age of a toddler
         (2) Demonstrates some understanding of speech and response
         (3) May respond to routines and repetitive actions but requires complete supervision and custodial care
      d) Profound (IQ below 20-25)
         (1) Achieves the mental age of an infant
         (2) Some sensorimotor capacity, but the child requires complete care and protection

B. Assessment
 1. Assess physical growth parameters and developmental tasks.
 2. Assess psychosocial parameters.
 3. Perform a cognitive assessment to determine mental age; compare the findings with the child's chronologic age.
 4. Use multiple tests to avoid making an assessment based on a test that fails to recognize the child's strengths.
 5. Arrange at least two testing sessions (determination of mental retardation is made over time).
 6. Determine family genetics and assess the home environment.
 7. Identify chronic conditions that could have interfered with learning and development.

C. Interventions
 1. Support the optimal development of the child.
 2. Help the parents mourn the loss of the wished-for child.
 3. Set realistic, reachable short-term goals; break tasks into small steps to encourage their successful accomplishment.
 4. Help the parents avoid frustration; the child's achievements will come slowly.
 5. Use behavior modification, if applicable.
 6. Stimulate and communicate at the child's mental age rather than chronologic age.
 7. Provide a safe environment.
 8. Mainstream daily routines to promote normalcy.
 9. Educate using effective adaptive teaching strategies.
 10. Teach self-care skills.

VI. Cerebral palsy (CP)

A. Introduction
 1. CP is a neuromuscular disorder resulting from damage to or aberrant structure of the brain area that controls motor function.
   a) It is caused by trauma (hemorrhage); anoxia before, during, or after birth; or infection.
   b) It is most commonly seen in children born prematurely.
 2. CP is a nonprogressive disorder.
 3. Disabilities associated with CP are as follows:
   a) Abnormal muscle tone and coordination (the most common problem associated with CP)
   b) Mental retardation of varying degrees in 18% to 50% (most children with CP have at least a normal IQ but cannot demonstrate it on standardized tests)

   c) Speech, vision, or hearing disturbances
   d) Dental anomalies
   e) Seizures
   f) Poor self-image and self-esteem

B. Assessment

 1. Assess for signs and symptoms of spastic CP; hypertonicity with poor posture control, leg scissoring, persistent primitive reflexes, altered quality of speech, poor coordination, and persistent muscle contraction (resulting in contractures).

 2. Assess for signs and symptoms of dyskinetic-athetotic CP; abnormal, constant, involuntary wormlike movements that disappear during sleep and increase with stress, especially affecting the facial muscles; decreased ability on fine motor skills; and no contractures.

 3. Assess for signs and symptoms of ataxic CP: poor equilibrium and muscle coordination, and an unsteady wide-based gait.

 4. Assess for signs and symptoms of rigid CP; simultaneous contraction of the contracting and extensor muscles, resulting in resistance to movement, diminished reflexes, and severe contractures.

 5. Assess for difficulty sucking in the newborn period.

C. Interventions

 1. Enable the child to attain optimal developmental level by assisting with locomotion, communication, and educational opportunities.

 2. Increase caloric intake for the child with increased motor function.

 3. Make food easy to manage; decrease stress during mealtimes.

 4. Provide a safe environment (for example, with protective headgear or bed pads).

 5. Provide rest periods.

 6. Use range-of-motion exercises, if the child is spastic; maintain proper body alignment.

 7. Promote age-appropriate mental activities and incentives for motor development.

 8. Divide tasks into small steps.

 9. Refer the child for speech, nutrition, and physical therapy.

 10. Promote a positive self-concept.
   a) Give the child enough time to share thoughts.
   b) Use other communication devices if speech is impossible.

VII. Seizure disorder

A. Introduction
1. A seizure is a sudden, episodic involuntary alteration in consciousness, motor activity, behavior, sensation, or autonomic function (see Table 4).
    a) The nerve cells become hyperexcitable and surpass the seizure threshold.
    b) The neurons overfire without regard to stimuli or need.
2. Childhood epilepsy is a term used to describe two or more unprovoked seizures in childhood; many types of seizures and seizure disorders are classified under childhood epilepsy.

Table 4. Classification of seizures

Type	Description	Symptoms
I. Partial (beginning locally)	Localized to one area of the brain (but may progress to generalized)	
A. Simple partial seizure	Symptoms confined to one hemisphere of the brain	May have motor (change in posture or repetitive movement of a limb), autonomic, sensory, or psychic (hallucinations) symptoms; no impairment of consciousness
B. Complex partial seizure	Begins in one focal area of the brain but spreads to both hemispheres	May have only loss of consciousness or may also have automatisms; loss of consciousness
II. Generalized	Initial onset appears in both hemispheres	Bilateral motor activity; loss of consciousness
A. Absence (petit mal)	Sudden onset; lasts 5 to 10 seconds; can have 100 daily; precipitated by stress, hyperventilation, hypoglycemia, fatigue, differentiated from daydreaming	Loss of responsiveness but continued ability to maintain posture control and not fall. Symptoms may include twitching eyelids and lip smacking. No postictal symptoms
B. Myoclonic	Movement disorder (not a seizure) seen as child awakens or falls asleep; may be precipitated by touch or visual stimuli; focal or generalized; symmetric or asymmetric	No loss of consciousness. Sudden, brief, shocklike involuntary contraction of one muscle group

C. Clonic	Opposing muscles contract and relax alternately in rhythmic pattern; may occur in one limb more than others	Mucus production
D. Tonic	Muscles are maintained in continuous contracted state (rigid posture)	Variable loss of consciousness; pupils dilate; eyes roll up; glottis closes; possible incontinence; may foam at mouth
E. Tonic-clonic	Violent total body seizure	Aura; tonic first (20 to 40 seconds); clonic next; postictal symptoms
F. Atonic	Drop and fall attack; needs to wear protective helmet	Loss of posture tone
G. Akinetic	Sudden brief loss of muscle tone or posture	Temporary loss of consciousness
III. Miscellaneous		
A. Febrile	Seizure threshold lowered by elevated temperature; only one seizure per fever; common in 4% of the population under 5 when temperature is rapidly rising	Lasts less than 5 minutes; generalized, transient, and nonprogressive; does not generally result in brain damage; electroencephalogram is normal after 2 weeks; may occur only once or may recur
B. Status epilepticus	Prolonged or frequent repetition of seizures without interruption; results in anoxia, cardiac and respiratory arrest	Consciousness not regained between seizures; lasts more than 30 minutes

B. Assessment
1. Ask if the child experiences an aura (preictal), a peculiar sensation just before the seizure's onset (unusual tastes, feelings, odors, or visual sensations).
2. Determine the nature of the seizure: the muscles involved, their position, symmetry or asymmetry of movement, the child's level of consciousness (LOC) and respiratory status, and whether the child is continent or incontinent.
3. Determine the postictal response: whether the child is oriented to time and place or drowsy and uncoordinated immediately following a seizure.
4. Note an altered electroencephalogram.

C. Interventions
1. Pad the crib or bed for any child with a history of seizures.
2. Stay with the child during a seizure.
3. Do not try to interrupt the seizure; it is best to allow the child to seize without interfering unless the child is in an unsafe place or near potentially harmful objects.
   a) If necessary, move the child to a flat surface, away from objects, and out of danger.
4. Promote a patent airway.
   a) Do *not* place anything in or near the mouth.
   b) If child becomes cyanotic or hypoxemic, administer oxygen when the seizure ends and regular respirations resume.
   c) Place the child on their side to let saliva drain out and allow tongue to fall forward and open airway.
5. Record seizure activity.
   a) Note the time the seizure starts and ends.
   b) Note the movement or nature of the seizure.
      (1) Symmetric versus asymmetric
      (2) Movement versus staring
6. Administer seizure medications.
   a) Phenytoin (Dilantin) keeps neuron excitability below the seizure threshold; side effects include gum hyperplasia, hirsutism, ataxia, gastric distress, nystagmus, anemia, and sedation.
   b) Other seizure medications include phenobarbital, carbamazepine (Tegretol), and valproic acid (Depakote).
7. Monitor serum levels of anticonvulsant medications, such as phenytoin, to ensure therapeutic levels and prevent toxicity.

8. Diastat (Valium) per rectum may be ordered for treatment *during* a seizure.
9. Instruct patient and parents in all aspects of seizure control measures (see Table 5).

Table 5. Teaching tips: Seizure disorders

> **Be sure to include the following points in your teaching plan for the parents of a child with a seizure disorder:**
>
> - Type of seizure and possible cause, if known
> - Medication regimen, including dose, frequency, times of administration, and possible side effects
> - Safety measures during seizure
> - Compliance with follow-up laboratory tests and physician visits
> - Promotion of as normal a life as possible for the child
> - Reinforcement of positive self-image
> - Notification of the school and sports teams
> - Awareness of the state laws regarding driving a car

VIII. Increased intracranial pressure

A. Introduction
    1. Increased intracranial pressure (ICP) may be caused by inflammation, tissue enlargement, or increased fluid accumulation.
    2. A persistent increase in ICP destroys healthy brain tissue and alters mental function.

B. Assessment before the closure of cranial sutures (see Section IX, Hydrocephalus, in this chapter)

C. Assessment after the closure of cranial sutures
    1. Assess for nausea, vomiting, and headache.
    2. Assess and record vital signs.
        a) Note increased blood pressure, decreased pulse rate, and decreased respiratory rate.
        b) Signs can deteriorate to the point of respiratory and cardiac arrest.
    3. Assess for blurred vision, papilledema, and altered pupil reaction to light.
    4. Monitor for personality changes.
    5. Observe for and monitor seizures.

6. Assess for an altered LOC, with decreased attention span or lethargy.
7. Observe for altered motor skills, such as clumsiness and loss of balance.
8. Measure head circumference and compare with past measurements.

D. Interventions
1. Elevate the head of the bed slightly to decrease cerebral edema.
2. Administer an osmotic diuretic (such as mannitol) to decrease cerebral edema.
3. Administer corticosteroids to decrease brain inflammation.
4. Limit fluids to decrease blood volume, which will reduce cerebral edema; maintenance fluids may be kept at three-fourths usual IV + oral (PO) maintenance fluid therapy (see Chapter 11).
5. Monitor fluids and electrolytes.
6. Perform hyperventilation with a bag-valve-mask device, if ordered.
7. Monitor the child's LOC.

IX. Hydrocephalus

A. Introduction
1. Hydrocephalus is an increase in the amount of cerebrospinal fluid (CSF) in the ventricles and subarachnoid spaces of the brain.
2. It is caused either by obstruction to the flow of CSF in the ventricular system (noncommunicating hydrocephalus) or by impaired absorption of the CSF in the arachnoid space (communicating hydrocephalus).
   a) Causes of noncommunicating hydrocephalus include tumors, hemorrhage, or structural abnormalities.
   b) Causes of communicating hydrocephalus include scarring, congenital anomalies, or hemorrhage.
3. Arnold-Chiari malformation is the downward displacement of cerebellar components through the foramen magnum into the cervical spinal canal; it is common in hydrocephalus associated with spina bifida.

B. Assessment
1. Measure the child's head circumference; note a rapid increase.
2. Observe for full, tense, bulging fontanels.

      3. Check for widening suture lines.

      4. Observe for distended scalp veins.

      5. Assess for irritability or lethargy; the child has a decreased attention span.

      6. Note a high-pitched cry.

      7. Note the sunset sign (sclera visible above the iris).

      8. Observe the child's inability to support the head when upright.

      9. Percuss the skull; note the "cracked pot" sound.

     10. Perform transillumination of the skull (the light will reflect off of the opposite side of the skull).

C. Interventions status post shunt insertion

      1. Observe for signs of shunt blockage as evidenced by signs of increased ICP (increased head circumference and a full fontanel).

      2. Observe for signs of infection.

      3. If the caudal end of the shunt must be externalized because of infection, keep the bag at ear level to prevent an increase or decrease in ICP.

      4. Support the child's head when the child is upright.

      5. Provide proper skin care to the head; turn it frequently.

      6. Teach parents signs of increasing ICP.

X. Intraventricular hemorrhage (IVH)

A. Introduction

      1. IVH is the rupture of a part of the vascular network of the germinal matrix, resulting in bleeding in the brain.

      2. The bleed is classified in four stages according to severity and extent of hemorrhage.

      3. IVH is most commonly found in preterm infants of less than 32 weeks gestation.

      4. IVH is associated with birth asphyxia, respiratory distress, metabolic instabilities, and use of drugs, such as surfactant therapy.

B. Assessment

      1. Measure head circumference daily; note increases of 0.5 cm or greater.

      2. Assess fontanels every 8 hours for fullness or bulging; check for widening of suture lines.

      3. Assess for increased incidence of apnea, bradycardia, changes in muscle tone or activity; and unexplained drops in hemoglobin and hematocrit.

4. Anticipate computed tomography (CT) or magnetic resonance imaging (MRI) scans to confirm extent of hemorrhage.

C. Interventions

1. Prevent IVH from occurring by preventing fluctuations in cerebral blood pressure (ICP).

2. Decrease noxious environmental stimuli; decrease noise, lights, and handling.

3. Maintain head in midline position to prevent venous congestion that results in hydrostatic pressure changes and increased ICP.

4. Monitor and treat pain, as pain can impede venous return and increase ICP.

5. Support the family by teaching developmentally supportive interventions that prevent IVH or prevent it from worsening.

XI. Neural tube defects

A. Introduction

1. Neural tube defects are a group of related CNS birth defects that arise from inappropriate closure of the embryonic neural tube; each different type of neural tube defect varies in the severity of associated clinical symptoms.

2. Neural tube defects are multifactorial in origin, associated with a deficiency in maternal folic acid around the time of conception.

3. There are several types of neural tube defects classified according to the portion of the CNS involved:

   a) Anencephaly—a condition in which both cerebral hemispheres are absent; the brain stem and cerebellum may be present; the condition is incompatible with life. Many infants are stillborn or die within hours of birth; organ donation is a consideration among anencephalic infants who are born living.

   b) Encephalocele—a condition involving herniation of the brain through a defect in the skull resulting in a fluid-filled sac, sometimes with brain tissue inside.

   c) Meningocele—a condition involving the hernial protrusion of a saclike cyst containing meninges but not spinal cord.

      d) Myelomeningocele—a condition in which the posterior portion of the vertebral laminae fails to close anywhere along the spinal cord, resulting in a protruding sac containing CSF, meninges, and a portion of the spinal cord; it is the most common type of spina bifida.

        (1) The failure occurs at 3 to 4 weeks' gestation.

        (2) Multiple handicaps can result because the spinal nerves are in the sac rather than in the spinal column.

        (3) Surgical correction usually occurs within 48 hours of birth.

  4. The defects can be found early in gestation; the amniotic fluid will contain high levels of alpha fetoprotein from the leaking CSF.

B. Assessment for spina bifida

  1. Check for leakage from the sac.

  2. Check for infection around the sac.

  3. Assess for signs and symptoms of CNS infection.

  4. Assess for motor activity below the sac.

  5. Measure the head circumference to establish baseline data.

  6. Assess bowel and bladder function and patterns.

C. Interventions (preoperative)

  1. Provide emotional support to the parents; be aware that surgery usually occurs 24 to 48 hours after birth.

  2. Prevent trauma by keeping pressure off the sac; keep the child on one side with the knees flexed or on the abdomen.

  3. Institute measures to keep the sac free of infection; avoid contamination from urine or stool.

  4. Prevent the sac from drying; cover it with saline-soaked sterile dressings.

D. Assessment (postoperative)

  1. Note the degree of leg movement in response to discomfort.

  2. Note the degree of sensitivity to touch below the level of the lesion; paralysis is possible.

  3. Observe for clubfoot.

  4. Observe for dribbling of urine, distended bladder, or the involuntary release of stool, which may indicate a neurogenic bladder and bowel.

  5. Observe for signs of increased ICP, possibly related to scarring of the spinal area and reduced absorptive space; measure head circumference.

  6. Note if the child is meeting developmental milestones.

E. Interventions (postoperative)
1. Provide routine postoperative care.
2. Provide thorough skin care if paralysis occurs; place child on sheepskin.
3. Provide orthopedic appliances, if necessary.
4. Prevent constipation.
5. Promote range of motion.
6. Teach clean intermittent catheterization.
7. Be aware of an increased incidence of latex allergies in this population.

XII. Meningitis

A. Introduction
1. Meningitis, an inflammation of the meninges, is caused by viral or bacterial agents and transmitted by the spread of droplets; organisms enter the blood from the nasopharynx or the middle ear.
2. The condition is common in infants and toddlers; its incidence is greatly decreased with the administration of *Haemophilus influenzae* type B vaccine.

B. Assessment
1. Note seizures.
2. Observe for signs of increased ICP: vomiting, irritability.
   a) Infants and young toddlers may exhibit a high-pitched cry, bulging fontanel, and poor feeding.
   b) Older children and adolescents may exhibit nuchal rigidity, headache.
3. Assess for abnormal postures such as
   a) Opisthotonos (hyperextension of the neck and spine), which may be present later in the course of illness
   b) Brudzinski's sign (the child will flex the knees and hips in response to passive neck flexion).
4. Observe for a petechial or purpuric rash, which is associated with particular types of bacterial infection.
5. Check ear drainage for CSF; the presence of CSF will give positive glucose results.
6. Note that lumbar puncture will show increased CSF pressure, cloudy color, increased white blood cells and protein counts, and a decreased glucose count if the meningitis is caused by bacteria.

    C.   Interventions

        1.   Institute seizure precautions.

        2.   Isolate the child for at least 24 hours after antibiotic therapy begins.

        3.   Assess the child's neurologic status frequently to monitor for increased ICP.

        4.   Provide a dark and quiet environment.

        5.   Keep the child flat in bed.

        6.   Move the child gently.

        7.   Administer parenteral antibiotics.

XIII.   Brain tumor

    A.   Introduction

        1.   Brain tumors are the second most prevalent type of cancer in children.

        2.   The condition is usually diagnosed when the child is between ages 5 and 10.

        3.   Almost two thirds of brain tumors in children are infratentorial, commonly involving the cerebellum or brain stem.

        4.   Gliomas are the most common brain tumors in children; they include medulloblastoma, astrocytoma, ependymoma, and craniopharyngioma.

        5.   Prognosis varies based on the type and location of the tumor.

    B.   Assessment

        1.   Symptoms stem from the tumor's pressure on adjacent neural tissues and/or on flow of CSF.

        2.   The young child is typically difficult to diagnose because of the elasticity of the skull and normally poor coordination.

        3.   ICP may increase.

        4.   Alterations in neurologic function, especially visual acuity and behavior changes, may occur, including a decline in school performance.

        5.   Headache, commonly an initial sign, usually occurs in the early morning on arising and during sneezing, coughing, and straining.

        6.   Vomiting, hypotonia, posturing, seizures, and altered vital signs may occur.

        7.   Other common signs and symptoms include ataxia (uncoordinated gait), cranial nerve palsies, anorexia, head tilt, nystagmus, decreased reflexes, vertigo, and a change in dexterity.

8. Assess for signs and symptoms of craniopharyngioma: pressure on the pituitary resulting in diabetes insipidus, visual problems, difficulty regulating body temperature, altered growth patterns, and altered CSF pressure.

C. Interventions (preoperative)
1. Prepare the child for a CT or MRI scan.
2. Prepare the child for radiotherapy prior to tumor removal, in an attempt to shrink the tumor.
3. Advise the child and parents to expect facial edema and hair loss from chemotherapy.

D. Interventions (postoperative)
1. Position the child on the nonoperative side to minimize pressure and prevent the brain from shifting into the space vacated by the tumor.
2. Make sure the child lies flat on either side if surgery was infratentorial to maintain a steady ICP; elevate the head of the bed slightly if surgery was supratentorial to promote venous drainage.
3. Monitor vital signs; check the pupils and report any inequality or sluggishness.
4. Maintain proper alignment; logroll if ordered.
5. Assess the child's LOC and ease of arousal; note any changes indicative of increasing ICP and report immediately.
6. Relieve eye edema with cold compresses; lubricate the eyes to prevent corneal irritation.
7. Prevent increased ICP by telling the child to avoid straining for stool or coughing forcefully.
8. Initiate seizure precautions.
9. Administer vasopressin (Pitressin) to treat diabetes insipidus for craniopharyngioma and replace lost fluid as ordered.

XIV. Head injuries

A. Introduction
1. Head injuries are a common cause of death in children older than age 1.
2. The extent of the brain injury is directly related to the force of impact.
3. An epidural, intracranial hemorrhage is bleeding into the spaces between the dura mater and the skull.
4. A subdural hemorrhage is bleeding between the dura mater and the arachnoid layer of the meninges.

5. A concussion is a transient state of neurologic dysfunction caused by a jarring of the brain; it is the most common head injury.

6. A skull fracture may be linear (simple), depressed (depression of a bone toward the brain), or basilar (at the skull base).

B. Assessment

1. For an epidural injury, assess for a recent history of head trauma with or without loss of consciousness; note increasing headaches, a decreasing LOC, contralateral hemiparesis, and bradycardia.

2. For a subdural injury, assess for any type of head trauma, such as from falls, accident, or abuse.

3. For a concussion, note the child's LOC and memory of the accident.

4. Assess for signs and symptoms of ICP.

5. Perform frequent neurologic assessments to determine quality of reflexes, pupillary reflex, and LOC using the Glasgow Coma Scale score (see Table 6).

6. Assess vital signs frequently.

7. Prepare for a CT scan.

8. Check ear or nose drainage for glucose (CSF tests positive for glucose).

9. Note behavioral changes, such as aggression, withdrawal, or irritability; watch for alterations in sleep patterns, gait, or school performance (for more information about assessing a head injury, see Table 7).

Table 6. Glasgow Coma Scale score and points

Eye-opening response:
spontaneous (4); to verbal commands or speech (3); to pain only (2); no response (1)

Verbal response:
oriented [for infant: coos/babbles (5); confused conversation, but able to answer questions [for infant: irritable/cries] (4); inappropriate words [for infant: cries to pain] (3); incomprehensible speech [for infant: moans/grunts] (2); no response (1)

Motor response:
obeys commands for movement (6); purposeful movement to painful stimulus (5); withdraws in response to pain (4); flexion in response to pain (decorticate posturing) (3); extension response in response to pain (decerebrate posturing) (2); no response (1)

Scores:
Severe head injury = 8 or less
Moderate head injury = 9-12
Mild head injury = 13-15

Table 7. Decision tree: Assessing a head injury

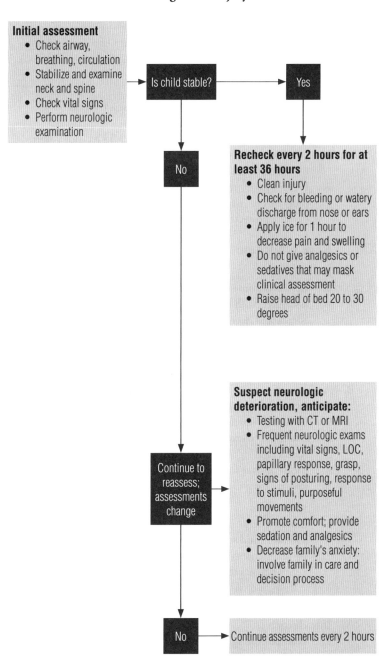

Initial assessment
- Check airway, breathing, circulation
- Stabilize and examine neck and spine
- Check vital signs
- Perform neurologic examination

Is child stable?

Yes

No

Recheck every 2 hours for at least 36 hours
- Clean injury
- Check for bleeding or watery discharge from nose or ears
- Apply ice for 1 hour to decrease pain and swelling
- Do not give analgesics or sedatives that may mask clinical assessment
- Raise head of bed 20 to 30 degrees

Suspect neurologic deterioration, anticipate:
- Testing with CT or MRI
- Frequent neurologic exams including vital signs, LOC, papillary response, grasp, signs of posturing, response to stimuli, purposeful movements
- Promote comfort; provide sedation and analgesics
- Decrease family's anxiety: involve family in care and decision process

Continue to reassess; assessments change

No

Continue assessments every 2 hours

C. Interventions
1. Prepare for surgical evaluation of the blood clot and ligation of the bleeding vessel, if necessary.
2. Promote bed rest and limit unnecessary body movements; slightly elevate the head of the bed.
3. Initiate seizure precautions.
4. Provide a quiet environment.
5. Awaken the child every 2 hours to assess for LOC.
6. Monitor fluid status carefully.
   a) Maintain clear liquids until the child has not vomited for at least 6 hours.
   b) Restrict fluids as needed to decrease ICP.
7. Prevent injury through family and community teaching programs to stress child safety (bicycle helmets, car restraining devices, protective skating and athletic equipment).

XV. Reye syndrome

A. Introduction
1. Reye syndrome is a disorder of toxic encephalopathy associated with fatty changes in the liver; there are cerebral edema and decreased LOC.
2. Reye syndrome is associated with viral infections such as varicella and influenza infection, particularly when combined with the administration of salicylates found in aspirin.

B. Assessment
1. Assess for signs and symptoms of ICP.
2. Perform frequent neurologic assessments to determine quality of reflexes, pupillary reflex, and LOC.
3. Assess vital signs frequently.
4. Monitor liver function test results.
5. Prepare for a CT scan.

C. Interventions
1. Initiate seizure precautions.
2. Monitor fluid status carefully; restrict intake to two-thirds IV maintenance fluid therapy (see Chapter 11).
3. Teach parents to avoid aspirin in children under 16 years.

XVI. Lead poisoning (plumbism)

A. Introduction
1. Lead poisoning (plumbism) is defined as the presence of blood lead levels (BLL) ≥10 µg/dl.

2. Lead poisoning occurs in children through ingestion of lead in lead-based paint chips or paint dust, contaminated drinking water from lead-based pipes, dust from lead ammunition, battery casings, collectible toys, and some jewelry.
3. Lead is carried by the RBCs and then deposited into the bone and tissues.
4. Lead is excreted in the urine and the bile; its half-life is 10 months.
5. Lead poisoning is a chronic condition that often goes unnoticed for extended periods of time; screening for risk factors is a key intervention.

B. Assessment
1. Observe for nausea, vomiting, anorexia, constipation, and abdominal pain.
2. Assess for symptoms of anemia: pallor, fatigue, tachycardia.
3. Assess for Fanconi-like syndrome of aminoaciduria, glucosuria, and hypophosphatemia.
4. Assess for neurologic signs of lead poisoning including behavioral changes, distractibility, learning difficulty, impaired intellect, and, in severe cases, signs of encephalopathy such as seizures and coma.
5. Assess for stunted growth in chronic lead poisoning.
6. Ask parents about a history of pica, the eating of nonfood substances, which is associated with lead poisoning.

C. Interventions
1. Provide lead screening at routine health visits; begin lead screening by one year of age.
2. Assist with obtaining serum lead level.
3. Administer IV lead chelation therapy, which binds with the lead and excretes it from the body.
4. Monitor for symptoms of lead toxicity.
5. Monitor fluid status.
   a) Promote fluid intake to promote excretion of lead.
   b) Monitor output to evaluate kidney function.
6. Perform serial urine testing as prescribed to evaluate kidney function and lead excretion.
7. Prevent further lead exposure.
   a) Provide parent and child education regarding lead poisoning (see Table 8).

Table 8. Lead poisoning prevention

- Prevent exposure to peeling, lead-based paint.
- If remodeling an older home, follow recommendations.
- Use only cold water from the faucet and allow it to run for 1 minute before using.
- Have water and soil tested.
- Do not store food in opened cans.
- Do not store food or drink from ceramicware or pottery containing lead.
- Ensure that children eat and drink adequate amounts of iron and calcium.

XVII. Migraine headaches

A. Overview
1. They are often accompanied by extreme sensitivity to light and sound, nausea and vomiting.
2. Migraines are three times more common in women than in men; affect 15% of population.
3. Some have an aura (visual disturbance, flashing lights, temporary loss of vision) before having a migraine.
4. A migraine headache typically lasts 4 to 72 hours.
5. They may be triggered by a lack of food or sleep, exposure to light, hormonal changes, anxiety, and stress.
6. They are believed to be inherited, but the etiology and pathophysiology are unknown.
7. The goal is to prevent attacks.

B. Interventions
1. Stress management strategies
2. Medications and hormones, especially related to the menstrual cycle

CHAPTER
15

Musculoskeletal Conditions

LEARNING OBJECTIVES

1. Determine the nursing interventions necessary for the child in a cast, traction, or brace.

2. Assess and plan care for the child with a musculoskeletal defect.

3. Describe how the musculoskeletal development from birth through adolescence predisposes the child to various orthopedic conditions.

I. Introduction

A. Bones and muscles grow and develop throughout childhood.

B. Bone length occurs in the epiphyseal plates at the ends of bones; when the epiphyses close, growth stops.
   1. Damage to the epiphyseal plates can disrupt bone growth.

C. Bone healing occurs much faster in the child than in the adult, because the child's bones are still growing.
   1. The younger the child, the faster the bone heals.
   2. Bone healing takes approximately 1 week for every year of life up to age 10.

D. Orthopedic anomalies may interfere with the function of other organ systems.

E. The most common fractures in the child are clavicular and greenstick.
   1. Clavicular fractures are common following vaginal birth, because the shoulders are the widest part of the body.
   2. Greenstick fractures of the long bones are related to the increased flexibility of the young child's bones; the compressed side bends and the tension side fractures.

II. General assessment of musculoskeletal deviation

A. Assess function in the affected part.
   1. Determine the range of motion.
   2. Note the amount of weight the child can bear.
   3. Assess gross and fine motor abilities.

B. Assess the quality of bone and tissue; check whether the correct amount of ossification is present when evaluated by X-ray.

C. Determine whether all bones are correctly aligned.

D. Determine whether musculoskeletal response is bilateral and equal.
   1. Note whether both arms and legs are used.
   2. Note whether muscle response is brisk and strong.

E. Assess for pain; note whether the child is guarding a body part.

F. Assess for muscle tone, degree of weakness, reflexes, pulses, sensation in affected extremities.

G. Determine the relationship of the child's body size and weight to the defect.

H. Note whether the child has an adequate and even spread of adipose tissue.

I. Note the child's autonomy and independence in terms of mobility and skills.

III. Common orthopedic interventions

A. Cast care (mostly for plaster casts)
   1. Turn the cast frequently to dry all sides; use palms to lift or turn a wet cast to prevent indentations.
   2. Expose as much of the cast to air as possible, but cover exposed parts.
   3. Be aware of discomfort to the child as chemical changes in the drying of a cast result in temperature extremes against the child's skin.
   4. After it is dry, maintain a dry cast; wetting the plaster cast will soften it and may cause skin irritation.
   5. Smooth out the cast's rough edges, and petal it with tape.
   6. Assess circulation.
      a) Note the color, pulses, sensation, movement, temperature, and edema of digits.
      b) Note the child's ability to wiggle the extremities without tingling or numbness.
   7. Assess for any drainage or foul odor from the cast.
   8. Prevent small objects or food from falling into cast.
   9. Do not use powder on the skin near the cast; it becomes a medium for bacteria when it absorbs perspiration.
   10. Before the cast is applied or removed, demonstrate the complete procedure on a doll, with the child's assistance.

B. Hip-spica cast (a body cast extending from mid-chest to the legs)
   1. The legs are abducted with a bar between them; never lift or turn the child with the crossbar.
   2. Perform cast care as listed above but with additional measures.
      a) Place a disposable diaper under the edges to prevent the cast from getting wet and soiled.
      b) Keep the cast level but on a slant, with the head of the bed raised.
         (1) Urine and stool will drain downward away from the cast.
         (2) A Bradford frame can be used for this purpose.

> > *c)* Use a mattress firm enough to support the cast; use pillows to support parts of the cast, if needed.
> >
> > *d)* Reposition the child frequently to avoid pressure on the skin and the bony prominences; check for pressure as the child grows.

C. Traction

1. Purpose is to decrease muscle spasms and realign and position bone ends.
2. There are different types of traction.

   a) Skin traction pulls indirectly on the skeleton by pulling on the skin via adhesive, moleskin, or an elastic bandage.

   b) Skeletal traction pulls directly on the skeleton via pins or tongs.

3. Keeping the child in alignment can be a challenge because of increased mobility and lack of understanding of the treatment.
4. Check that the weights hang free.
5. Check for skin irritation, infection at pin sites, and neurovascular response of the extremity.
6. Place on pressure-reducing surface (sheepskin, alternating pressure mattress, etc.).
7. Prevent constipation by increasing fluids and fiber.
8. Prevent respiratory congestion by promoting pulmonary hygiene using blowing games.
9. Provide pain relief, if necessary.
10. Provide developmental stimulation.
11. Use Bryant's traction.

    a) This is the only skin traction designed specifically for the lower extremities of the child under age 2; the child provides his or her own countertraction.

    b) Legs are to be kept straight and extend 90° toward the ceiling from the trunk; both legs are suspended even if only one is affected.

    c) The buttocks are kept slightly off the bed to ensure sufficient and continuous traction on the legs.

    d) Traction is often followed by the application of a hip-spica cast.

D. Braces

1. These appliances assist in mobility and posture and may be a plastic shell or a metal-hinged appliance.

2. Provide good skin care, especially at the bony prominences.
3. Check to ensure accurate fit as the child grows.
4. When applying full body braces to a child with spasticity, put the feet in first.
5. Chest braces used for scoliosis extend from the iliac crest of the pelvis to the axilla; they must be fitted individually.
6. Chest braces are worn up to 23 hours a day, removed only for bathing and swimming.
7. Chest braces are worn over a thin t-shirt.

IV. Clubfoot (talipes)

A. Overview
   1. Clubfoot is a congenital disorder.
   2. The foot and ankle are twisted and cannot be passively manipulated into correct position.

B. Assessment
   1. Assess for talipes varus (inversion of the ankles, with the soles of the feet facing each other).
   2. Assess for talipes valgus (eversion of the ankles, with the feet turning out).
   3. Assess for talipes equinus (plantar flexion, as if pointing one's toes).
   4. Assess for talipes calcaneus (dorsiflexion, as if walking on one's heels).
   5. Assess for a combination of positions; most cases are equinovarus.

C. Interventions
   1. Assist with the application of a series of foot casts to gradually stretch and realign the angle of the foot.
   2. Perform passive range-of-motion exercises.
   3. Ensure that shoes fit correctly.
   4. If corrective devices are ordered, have the child keep the devices on as much as possible; stress the importance of this to the parents.
   5. Prepare for surgery, if necessary.

V. Congenital hip dysplasia/dislocated hip

A. Overview

1. Abnormal development of the head of the femur and acetabulum; present at birth and more common in females than males

2. Occurs when the head of the femur is still cartilaginous and the acetabulum is shallow; the head of the femur comes out of the hip socket

3. May be from the fetal position in utero, a breech delivery, genetic predisposition, or laxity of the ligaments

4. Occurs in varying degrees of dislocation, from partial subluxation to complete

5. Can affect one or both hips

B. Assessment

1. Assess for restricted abduction of the hips.

2. Assess for Ortolani's click.

   a) May be felt by the fingers at the hip area as the femur head snaps out and back in the acetabulum

   b) Palpable during examination with the child's legs flexed and abducted

3. Note the appearance of a shortened limb on the affected side (telescoping) when the child is supine.

4. Note asymmetrical skinfolds in gluteus from telescoping and dislocation.

   a) The affected side exhibits an increased number of folds on the posterior thigh when the child is supine with the knees bent.

   b) Flattened buttocks appear on the affected side when the child is prone.

5. Assess for Trendelenburg's sign in older children (when the child stands on the affected leg, the opposite pelvis dips to maintain erect posture).

C. Interventions

1. Be aware that the goal of treatment is to enlarge and deepen the socket by pressure.

2. Gently stretch and maintain the legs in an abducted position for at least 3 months, using triple-cloth diapering, casting, or a Pavlik harness, which keeps the hips and knees flexed and the hips abducted.

3. Use Bryant's traction if the acetabulum does not deepen.

4. Be aware that the older child may need a hip-spica cast or corrective surgery.

VI. Legg-Calvé-Perthes disease

A. Overview
1. Ischemic aseptic necrosis of the head of the femur, resulting in degenerative changes from a disturbance of circulation to the femoral capital epiphysis
2. Affects the preschool and school-age child

B. Assessment
1. Review the child's history for a limp and hip pain or pain referred to the knee.
2. Assess for limited hip motion.
3. Be aware that the disease must be differentiated from synovitis.

C. Interventions
1. Tell the parents that treatment lasts 2 to 3 years as revascularization occurs.
2. Be aware that the younger the child, the better the prognosis for recovery and the natural remodeling of the joint.
3. Tell the parents that the child must avoid weight bearing until reossification occurs; this relieves pressure from the head of the femur and increases blood flow to the area, thus preventing degeneration.
4. Be aware that bed rest with traction is followed by an abduction brace.

VII. Slipped capital femoral epiphysis

A. Overview
1. The proximal femoral epiphysis is displaced.
2. Growth hormones weaken the epiphyseal plate in the hip joint.
3. Displacement occurs in the adolescent who is actively growing or is overweight.

B. Assessment
1. Review the child's history for a limp.
2. Ask about pain in the groin or knee.
3. Note that the foot turns outward during gait; there is limited internal rotation and hip abduction.

C. Interventions
1. Prepare for possible skeletal traction, which may be followed by a hip-spica cast.

2. Prepare for possible surgical stabilization and immobilization of the hip with a pin.
3. Teach the obese child and the parents that weight loss will decrease stress on the bones.
4. Continuously assess the opposite hip since the condition may recur there; teach the parents to maintain this assessment.

VIII. Scoliosis

A. Overview
1. Lateral curvature of the spine
    a) Kyphosis is protrusion/convex angulation of the spine or "humpback."
    b) Lordosis is accentuation of the lumbar curvature of the spine or "swayback"; it is normal in toddlers.
2. Commonly identified at puberty and throughout adolescence, especially among females
3. Ceases to progress when bone growth ceases
4. Can be nonstructural/functional/postural
    a) A nonprogressive C curve may exist from some other deformity, such as unequal leg length
    b) When the child bends forward at the waist to touch toes, the curve in the spinal column disappears.
    c) Treatment may be shoe lifts, postural exercises, or corrective lenses, if the problem is caused by poor vision resulting in a head tilt
5. Is structural and progressive in most cases

B. Assessment of structural scoliosis
1. A progressive S curve with a primary and compensatory curvature can be seen when the child is standing; this can result in spinal and rib changes on X-ray.
2. When the child bends forward with the knees straight and the arms hanging down toward the feet, the spinal curve fails to straighten.
3. The hips, ribs, shoulders, and shoulder blades are asymmetrical.
4. X-rays assist in the diagnosis.
5. The curve often worsens with increased growth.
6. Assess for skin irritation by braces.

C. Interventions
1. Teach the child stretching exercises for the spine.
2. Expect possible prolonged bracing, usually a chest brace; assure good skin care is provided.

3. Be aware that skin traction or halo femoral traction may be used.
4. Be aware that electrical stimulation may be used for mild to moderate curvatures.
5. Provide emotional support to help the child feel attractive while wearing the brace.
6. Be aware that correction may involve spinal fusion with bone from the iliac crest.
   a) Instrumentation of the spine with rods and screws to attain alignment may be needed when curves fail to respond to orthotic treatment.
   b) Postoperatively, assure that child is turned by logrolling.
   c) Postoperatively, maintain bed in flat position and maintain correct body alignment.

IX. Osteogenesis imperfecta

A. Overview
1. It is an autosomal dominant disorder of the connective tissue, involving bones, ligaments, and sclera, with different degrees of presentation.
2. The absence of normal adult collagen results in brittle bones, which are easily fractured; bone fragility begins to ease with puberty.
3. Symptoms may be confused with those of child abuse; this condition is no one's fault.

B. Assessment
1. Review the child's history for frequent fractures with abnormal healing (bones thickened, curved, or otherwise altered in shape with repeated improper healing).
2. Assess for impaired growth and development.
3. Observe for blue-tinged sclera and thin skin.
4. Check for bluish-gray teeth from hypoplasia of dentin.
5. Assess for deafness from otosclerosis.
6. Be aware that spinal deformities often occur as the child reaches maturity.
7. Be aware that immobility for the healing of one fracture may predispose the child to another.

C. Interventions
1. Provide gentle handling in all child care activities.
2. Be aware that pins may be used instead of casts.
3. Provide a padded and soft environment.

X. Juvenile rheumatoid arthritis (JRA)

A. Overview
   1. It is an autoimmune disease of the connective tissue characterized by chronic inflammation of the synovia and possible joint destruction.
   2. Genetic predisposition appears to be passed by HLA.
   3. Episodes may recur with remissions and exacerbations.

B. Pauciarticular JRA
   1. Asymmetrical involvement of fewer than five joints, usually affecting large joints such as the knees, ankles, and elbows
   2. May lead to iridocyclitis (scarring and adhesions of the iris and ciliary body), resulting in cataracts and loss of vision

C. Polyarticular JRA
   1. Symmetrical involvement of five or more joints, especially hands and weight-bearing joints, such as hips, knees, and feet
   2. Involvement of the temporomandibular joint, which may cause earache; involvement of the sternoclavicular joint, which may cause chest pain

D. Systemic disease with polyarthritis
   1. This involves the lining of the heart and lungs, blood cells, and abdominal organs.
   2. Exacerbations may last for months.
   3. Fever, rash, and lymphadenopathy may occur.

E. Assessment
   1. Assess for signs and symptoms of inflammation around the joints.
   2. Check for stiffness, pain, and guarding of the affected joints.
   3. Note that blood tests show an elevated erythrocyte sedimentation rate, a positive antinuclear antibody, and the presence of rheumatoid factor (positive test results are not present in many children with the condition).
   4. Assist in the slit-lamp evaluation for iridocyclitis.

F. Interventions
   1. Teach the child that stress, climate, and genetics can influence exacerbations.
   2. Administer low-dose corticosteroids or nonsteroidal anti-inflammatory drugs, such as naproxen and ibuprofen; low-dose methotrexate may be used as a second-line medication.

3. Assist with exercise and range-of-motion activities.
4. Apply warm compresses or encourage the child to take a warm bath in the morning.
5. Apply splints.
6. Stress the need for preventive eye care.
7. Provide assistance devices, if necessary; encourage the normal performance of daily activities.
    a) May require additional time to perform activities of daily living, especially upon awakening.

XI. Duchenne's muscular dystrophy

A. Overview
   1. One of many muscular deterioration disorders that progress throughout childhood
   2. Genetic; sex-linked recessive; occurs only in males
   3. Absence of a protein in the muscles

B. Assessment
   1. Assess for delayed motor development.
   2. Note the disorder's progression.
      a) Begins with pelvic girdle weakness, indicated by a waddling gait and falling
      b) Proceeds to muscle weakness and wasting; progresses to the shoulder girdle; lordosis may occur
   3. Observe for Gower's sign (use of hands to push self up from floor).
   4. Note decreased ability to perform self-care activities.
   5. Assess for eventual contractures and muscle hypertrophy.
   6. Note fibrous degeneration and fatty deposits on muscle biopsy.
   7. Assess for cardiac or pulmonary failure.

C. Interventions
   1. Ensure that the child remains as active and independent as possible.
   2. Perform range-of-motion exercises.
   3. Apply splints as necessary.
   4. Provide emotional support to the parents; initiate genetic counseling.

XII. Hernias and hydroceles

A. Overview

1. Hernias are a muscle weakness causing the protrusion of an organ through the abnormal musculature.

   a) Umbilical hernia is failure of the umbilical muscles to close at birth resulting in protrusion of the omentum and intestine through the navel.

   b) Inguinal canal hernia is weakness where the testes descended from the abdomen to the scrotum; failure of the proximal portion of the inguinal canal to atrophy resulting in protrusion.

2. An irreducible hernia is a protrusion that will not return to its normal position.

3. An incarcerated hernia occurs when the abdominal contents become trapped and irreducible.

4. A strangulated hernia occurs when the herniated intestines become twisted and edematous resulting in intestinal obstruction and ischemia.

5. A hydrocele is a collection of peritoneal fluid in the scrotal sac; it may be communicating or noncommunicating.

B. Assessment

1. Assess for an increase in the size of the lump as the child strains, coughs, or cries.

2. Note that the condition is usually present without pain.

3. Observe for symptoms of incarceration (pain, irritability, intestinal obstruction due to the loop of bowel becoming occluded so that solids cannot pass).

C. Interventions

1. Tell parents that home measures such as belly bands and abdominal binders are not effective.

2. Remember that the abdominal muscles often strengthen as the child grows, and the hernia and hydrocele may resolve without treatment.

3. Nonoperative reduction of an incarcerated hernia is attempted before surgical repair, with the contents of the hernia gently manipulated back into the abdomen followed by application of an ice pack.

4. Be aware that if the hernia does not resolve, surgical intervention may be required (herniorrhaphy); this is usually done on an outpatient basis.

CHAPTER
16

Dermatologic Conditions

LEARNING OBJECTIVES

1. Assess and plan care for the child with a rash.
2. Differentiate between contact dermatitis and infectious dermatitis.
3. Discuss the nursing interventions for the child with burns.

I. Rashes

A. Overview
1. The skin of children is thinner and more sensitive than that of adults.
2. Apparent birthmarks in the newborn result from the sensitivity of the infant's skin, the incomplete migration of skin cells, or clogged pores.
3. Heat aggravates most skin rashes and increases pruritus (itching); coolness decreases pruritus.
4. Most skin rashes are macular, papular, or vesicular.
   a) Macular rash: a flat rash with color changes in circumscribed areas
   b) Papular rash: raised solid lesions with color changes in circumscribed areas
   c) Vesicular rash: small, raised circumscribed lesions filled with clear fluid
5. Urticaria is also known as hives and may accompany other symptoms of allergy.

B. Assessment
1. Describe the size, shape, type, location, warmth, and color of the rash.
2. Note whether the erythema (redness) is blotchy or in discrete areas.
3. Assess the distribution of the rash (linear, circular, general).
4. Note whether the rash is dry or oozing; note if hemorrhage or petechiae are present.
5. Does the rash "come and go?"
6. When did the rash first appear and where?
7. Note tenderness, pain, or pruritus; note any change in sensation.
8. Check the status of the hair and hair shafts.
9. Review the child's history for allergies, contactants, new foods ingested, new clothes, wearing of others' clothes, medications taken, or recent hikes in the woods.
10. Evaluate the type of soaps used for laundry and body; keep the use of soap to a minimum.
11. Assess for other signs of systemic illness.
12. Has the child traveled anywhere recently?

C. Interventions
1. Apply cool, soothing soaks, give baths with added baking soda, or dab site with calamine lotion (but limit baths to once a day).
2. Administer antipruritics; give antihistamines if the rash is from an allergy.
3. Distract the child and provide projects that make use of the hands.
4. Keep the affected area clean and pat it dry; expose the affected area to air.
5. Do not apply powder or cornstarch, as they encourage bacterial growth.
6. Do not use commercially prepared diaper wipes on broken skin unless they are alcohol free, as they will irritate and burn.
7. Apply moisturizer to wet skin.
8. Prevent the spread of infection.
   a) Teach good hand washing.
   b) Keep weeping lesions covered.
   c) Teach the child not to share combs or hats and not to scratch.
9. Prevent secondary infections by cutting the child's nails and applying mittens and elbow restraints, if needed.
10. Suggest light, loose, nonirritating clothing, such as cotton.
11. A humidifier in the home may improve dry skin.

II. Contact dermatitis: Diaper rash

A. Overview
1. It is related to the moist, warm environment contained by a plastic diaper lining.
2. Condition may be caused by clothing dyes or the soaps used to wash diapers.
3. Condition may be caused by body soaps, bubble baths, tight clothes, and wool or rough clothing.
4. Skin may be further irritated by acidic urine and stool or the formation of ammonia in the diaper.

B. Assessment
1. Look for the characteristic bright red maculopapular rash in the diaper area.
2. Note irritability, since the rash is painful and warm.
3. Note any bleeding or "weeping."

C. Interventions
1. Keep the diaper area clean and dry.
   a) Change the diaper immediately after the child voids or stools.
   b) Wash the area with mild soap and water.
2. Keep the area open to the air without plastic bed linings, if possible.
3. Apply vitamin A and D skin cream or other creams for diaper rash to help skin heal.

III. Contact dermatitis: Poison ivy

A. Overview
1. Poisonous oil on the plant leaf causes a delayed hypersensitivity (T-cell) response; trauma to the leaves releases the sap, which is dragged across the skin.
2. The rash appears 5 to 21 days after the first exposure but 1 to 2 days after subsequent contact.
3. Oils that remain on the clothes and skin are contagious to others; the eruptions are *not* a source of infection and will *not* spread the disease.
4. Animals may carry the oils to humans.

B. Assessment
1. Assess for pruritus.
2. Observe for red, localized streaks that precede vesicles; vesicles break and fluid crusts.

C. Interventions
1. Wash the oils from the skin with soap and water as soon as possible after contact to prevent absorption through the skin.
2. Do not touch other body parts until the area has been cleansed.
3. Carefully wash resin out of clothes.
4. Apply calamine lotion and administer antihistamines, if ordered.
5. Prevent secondary infection from scratching.

IV. Impetigo

A. Overview
1. A superficial infection of the skin caused by group A β-hemolytic streptococci; may also be due to staphylococci

2. Highly contagious until all lesions are healed
   a) The infection is spread by direct contact.
   b) The incubation period is 2 to 5 days after contact.
3. Commonly seen on the face and extremities, but may be spread on other parts of the body by scratching
4. Can be spread by biting and stinging insects
5. Common in children ages 2 to 5 years

B. Assessment
   1. Assess for a macular rash that progresses to a papular and vesicular rash, which oozes and forms a moist, honey-colored crust.
   2. Assess for pruritus.
   3. Ask about bug bites.
   4. Ask about others who may have the same rash.

C. Interventions
   1. Apply moist soaks to soften the lesions; remove the crusts gently three to four times a day and wash the area.
   2. Cover the child's hands, if necessary, to prevent secondary infection; cut the child's nails.
   3. Cover the lesions to prevent their spread.
   4. Administer antibiotics for their full course.
   5. Explain the infectious nature of the condition to parents.
      a) Patient should use separate towels and linens.

V. Eczema

A. Overview
   1. A general term used to describe a condition of redness, scaling vesicles, and crusting
   2. May present as allergic contact or atopic dermatitis or as a reaction to stress
   3. Usually occurs as a chronic relapsing pruritic condition
   4. Often resolves by adulthood, but other forms of allergies may appear, such as asthma

B. Assessment
   1. Review the child's history of allergies.
   2. Note erythema, edema, and weeping vesicles, with the most common sites being the warmer and wetter areas (antecubital and popliteal spaces), thighs, neck, hands, cheeks, scalp, and groin.
   3. If chronic, skin pattern may change over time and thicken (lichenification) with deeper skin lines.

    C.   Interventions

        1.   The goal is to break the inflammatory and itch-scratch cycle.

        2.   Avoid wool and other itchy fabrics against the skin.

        3.   Apply steroid creams and topical immunomodulators.

        4.   Administer oral antihistamines.

        5.   Prevent secondary infections.

VI. Cutaneous fungal infections/ringworm

    A.   Overview

        1.   Tinea refers to an infection with a fungus.

        2.   Tinea capitis involves the hair.

           a)   Common in school-age children

           b)   Transmitted by personal contact and occasionally by pets

        3.   Tinea corporis or ringworm involves the trunk, extremities, and groin.

        4.   Tinea cruris is "jock itch"; it is not contagious to others.

        5.   Tinea pedis is "athlete's foot."

    B.   Assessment

        1.   Tinea capitis: scaling scalp or patchy hair loss

           a)   Organism invades the hair shaft; hair breaks off in affected area causing spotty areas of alopecia.

           b)   It spreads in a circular pattern.

        2.   Tinea cruris: in crural folds of the groin

           a)   Itching increases when child has been sweating after exercise or on warm days.

           b)   Inflammation occurs with continued wearing of occlusive clothing.

        3.   Tinea pedis: usually is interdigital (between toes)

           a)   Itching or pain in affected area

           b)   May have fissures between toes with underlying erythematous skin that may weep

        4.   Tinea corporis

           a)   Can be transferred from other body parts or from household contacts or from animals

           b)   May have one or more lesions

               (1)   Lesions may be annular (ring shaped), thus the name ringworm.

               (2)   Annular, scaling erythematous plaques with sharply marginated, indurated, and hyperkeratotic borders.

               (3)   Center of the ring may be clear.

               (4)   Ring may consist of vesicles.

C. Interventions
   1. Tinea capitis
      a) Apply oral and topical antifungal medications.
      b) Shampoo with Selsun Blue; have all household contacts do the same.
      c) Clean all contaminated objects to prevent reinfection.
   2. Tinea cruris
      a) Apply antifungal powders, creams, or lotions.
      b) Avoid tight-fitting clothing; wear loose underwear instead of briefs.
      c) Change underwear often, especially when the child is hot and sweaty.
      d) Shower after exercise and then apply the antifungal preparation.
      e) Avoid storing damp clothing in a locker or gym bag; wash clothes after each wearing to avoid reinfection.
   3. Tinea pedis
      a) Wear shoes while showering in public facilities to prevent spread.
      b) Apply antifungal cream, powder, or spray.
   4. Tinea corporis
      a) Apply antifungal medications.
         (1) Creams should be applied to the lesion and the surrounding skin, since this fungus spreads outward.

VI. Candidiasis/thrush

A. Overview
   1. *Candida albicans* is a yeastlike fungus normally found in the gastrointestinal tract and vagina and on the skin.
   2. It tends to grow in moist warm areas.
   3. It is usually found on mucous membranes and in folds of skin; commonly seen in obese individuals.
   4. Condition can occur as a result of oral antibiotic therapy.
   5. Hyperglycemia can predispose one to *Candida* infection.

B. Assessment
   1. Child may complain of itching, burning, and irritation.
   2. In the mouth, condition appears as white plaques with an underlying bright red surface; lesions may extend to the esophagus.
   3. Skin lesions appear red and moist

C. Interventions
1. Administer oral antifungal suspensions for oral thrush.
2. Keep skin areas dry. Use creams/ointments that heal skin.
    a) Keep skin layers separated from each other by inserting a flat thin cloth in folds.
    b) Cool water or Burow's solution soaks are soothing.
    c) May suggest use of a blow-dryer after bathing to ensure drying of skin, but assure that the distance is far enough away to prevent burns
3. Wear loose-fitting cotton clothing.
4. Lower humidity in the home environment.

VII. Pediculosis/lice

A. Overview
1. Common in school-age children who share clothing and combs and who have close physical contact
2. Unrelated to the hygiene of the child or family
3. Caused by a blood-obligate parasite; the parasites must feed at least once a day (therefore they live close to the scalp)
4. Easily transmitted from person to person, but lice do not fly or jump
5. Rarely causes systemic disease
6. Three species
    a) Pediculosis capitis: head lice
    b) Pediculosis corporis: body lice
        (1) Is correlated with poor hygiene
        (2) Lives in clothing and bedding
    c) Pubic lice (sometimes called "crabs")
        (1) If seen in children, assess for sexual activity or abuse.
7. Life cycle of louse 23 to 30 days

B. Assessment
1. Assess for lice eggshell cases (nits) that look like white flecks attached firmly to the base of the hair shafts; they do not flake off as with dandruff. (Note: it is difficult to detect if the nits contain live lice; only those with live lice need to be treated. Those that are close to the scalp and camouflaged in color are usually live.)
2. Ask about intense pruritus of the scalp.
3. Assess for secondary infection from scratching.

C. Interventions
1. Use pyrethrins (Rid) or permethrin (Nix) shampoo.
   a) Carefully follow manufacturer's directions to avoid neurotoxicity.
2. After washing hair, remove nits with a fine-tooth comb.
3. Wash bed linens, hats, combs, brushes, and anything else in contact with the hair; reinfestation occurs easily.
4. Avoid head-to-head contact.
5. Do not share clothing, hats, towels, brushes, combs, hair accessories.

VIII. Scabies

A. Overview
1. Scabies is a contagious mite infestation.
2. It is usually contracted by close body contact with infected individual.
3. Mite burrows into skin and deposits eggs there; eggs hatch over 30 days and travel to skin (so the incubation is 1-2 months).

B. Assessment
1. Assess for intense itching, worse at night.
2. Assess for rash that affects between fingers, wrists, genitals, waist, buttocks, knees, elbows; does not usually affect the face.
3. Ask if others in the family have the same condition.
4. Observe skin for "burrows" that may be linear, curved, or S-shaped and may include macules, papules, or erythematous lines.

C. Interventions
1. Application of a scabicide (e.g., Elimite) is curative; apply to areas below the neck and leave on for 8 to 12 hours; then wash off.
2. Household contacts should also be treated.
3. Wash all clothing and linens in hot cycle; if articles cannot be washed, seal in a plastic bag for 3 weeks.

IX. Acne

A. Overview
1. Most common among adolescents from hormonal stimulation and an increase in sebaceous gland activity, plus the presence of bacteria that is normally on the skin, breaking down fatty acids

        a)   The narrow channel between the gland and the surface becomes plugged with sebum.

        b)   The follicles expand into comedones, or pimples.

   2.   Not caused by foods, poor hygiene, hairstyles, or emotions, although some of these factors can exacerbate the condition; may also be exacerbated by menses, sweating, wearing helmets, and cosmetics

   3.   Most common on the face, chest, and back

B.   Assessment

   1.   Assess for characteristic noninflammatory whiteheads (comedones that remain closed at the skin surface) on chest, face, neck, upper arms, and back.

   2.   Assess for characteristic noninflammatory blackheads (comedones exposed to air [not dirt] that change color as they oxidize).

   3.   Assess for any signs of inflammation.

   4.   Ask the youth how he or she cares for the acne.

C.   Interventions

   1.   Tell the youth to wash the face twice daily with soap and water.

   2.   Apply topical benzoyl peroxide; oral antibiotics may be recommended.

   3.   Encourage youth not to pick or squeeze eruptions, as this can lead to scarring.

   4.   Promote self-esteem.

   5.   Address the child's emotional concerns, and eliminate any factors known to exacerbate acne.

   6.   If Accutane is ordered, female patients need a pregnancy test and must be taught to use two methods of birth control from 1 month before to 1 month after the use of this drug because of the extreme teratogenic properties.

X. Burns

A.   Overview

   1.   Most pediatric burns occur in children under age 5.

   2.   Burns are the third largest cause of accidental death in children, after motor vehicle accidents and drowning.

   3.   Under age 3, most burns result from contact with hot liquids or electricity.

   4.   Older children are most commonly burned by flames.

   5.   The rule of nines has proved inaccurate for children because the head can account for 13% to 19% of body surface area; the legs account for 10% to 16%, depending on the age and size of the child.

B. Assessment
1. Assess for first-degree burn (partial thickness).
   a) Dry, painful, red skin with edema
   b) Looks like sunburn
2. Assess for second-degree burn (partial thickness).
   a) Moist weeping blisters with edema
   b) Very painful
3. Assess for third-degree burn (full thickness).
   a) Dry, pale, leathery skin
   b) Avascular without blanching or pain.
4. Assess for fluid shift from intravascular to interstitial compartments.
5. Assess for hypovolemia and symptoms of shock from fluid shift, including renal function.
6. Assess for infection due to altered skin integrity.
7. Assess for diuresis 2 to 5 days after the burn, as fluid shifts back.

C. Interventions
1. Maintain a patent airway.
2. For an immediate burn:
   a) Stop the burning process.
   b) Remove burning and hot clothing and jewelry.
   c) Do not put anything on the burn other than cool water; do not use ice.
   d) Cover with clean sheet to prevent heat loss.
3. Prevent and treat shock.
4. Monitor for fluid balance.
5. Relieve pain; do *not* give intramuscular injections because of inconsistent absorption of medication.
   a) Reassure child that pain is *not* punishment.
6. Care for the burn wound.
   a) Assist with debridement, although this is often done in the OR.
   b) Elevate the burned part.
   c) Apply thin layer of topical burn cream.
7. To prevent sunburn:
   a) Avoid sun exposure between 10 a.m. and 3 p.m. when the sun's rays are the strongest.
   b) Wear protective clothing.
   c) Wear sunscreen.

XI. Body piercing and tattooing

A. Overview
 1. Every part of the body can be pierced or tattooed.
 2. The goal is to prevent infection.
 3. Piercings take 4 weeks to 8 months for the piercing site to heal; the navel may take up to 1 year because of the increased irritation of the waistband and the warmth of the area resulting in increased risk of infection.

B. Assessment
 1. Assess for infection at the site (redness, edema, pain, heat, yellow or green drainage).
 2. Assess for an allergic reaction at the site (edema, pruritus).

C. Interventions
 1. Emphasize hand washing and keeping hands from piercing or tattoo site.
 2. Wash piercing site with antibacterial soap and water twice a day; do not use alcohol or hydrogen peroxide, as they interfere with healing.
 3. For oral piercings, rinse mouth with antiseptic mouthwash (without alcohol) after eating.
 4. For an infection at the site of a piercing, *do not remove jewelry* as this will result in an abscess; treat infection with the jewelry still in.
 5. For an allergic reaction to the pierced jewelry, remove the jewelry.
 6. For tattoos, apply a dressing only for the first few hours until the bleeding stops.
 7. Keep tattoos clean by washing with antibacterial soap and water twice daily and applying a thin coat of antibiotic ointment for a few days to prevent scabs and preserve artwork.
 8. For allergic reactions to particular tattoo colors, the treatment is to "retattoo" the site with a tattoo needle without dyes to allow the color to seep out of the skin, thus decreasing the reaction.
 9. For tattoos, avoid scratching, swimming, or hot tubs until the tattoo has healed.
 10. For tattoos, wear sunblock to prevent fading.

CHAPTER

17

Psychiatric and Psychological Conditions

LEARNING OBJECTIVES

1. Identify assessments and interventions for the child with autism.

2. Compare and contrast anorexia and bulimia.

3. Assess for behaviors of attention-deficit/hyperactivity disorder.

4. Recommend interventions for learning disabilities.

5. Plan interventions for the child with mental retardation.

6. Discuss the principles of a therapeutic relationship with children.

I. Therapeutic counseling

A. Goals are to impart knowledge, decrease stress, build self-esteem and self-confidence, learn conflict resolution, recognize what is normal, develop coping skills.

B. Focus on needs, experiences, feelings, ideas.

C. Have good listening skills, a genuine interest, empathy, acceptance, positive regard.

D. Be nonjudgmental; do not impart your value system.

E. Promote trust.

F. Suggest interventions that are age appropriate and culturally appropriate.

G. If promises are made, they must be kept; you cannot promise to keep a secret if it involves danger to the child or to others or if it involves abuse.

H. There must be congruence between what is said and what is done.

I. Observe body language, tone of voice, facial expressions.

J. Use lines like, "Tell me what it is like to…", "How do you suppose someone feels when…", "What scares you the most?" "If you had three wishes, what would they be?"

K. Make a concrete plan.

II. Child abuse

A. Introduction
1. Child abuse comprises intentional acts of physical, emotional, or sexual abuse of a child or neglect of the child.
2. Infants and toddlers are the most common victims of physical abuse; school-age and adolescent children are at a higher risk for emotional and sexual abuse.
3. Child abuse usually indicates a serious family dysfunction in communicating and coping; the child, the focal point of stress, usually becomes a scapegoat.
4. Child abuse may result from the parents' unrealistic expectations of the child's physical and psychosocial abilities.
5. Child abusers come from all social classes and educational backgrounds; about 10% have serious psychological disturbances.

        a)   Many child abusers were abused as children and may not know healthier ways to discipline a child or to show love.

        b)   Child abusers characteristically have low self-esteem, little confidence, and a low tolerance for frustration.

  6. Sexual abuse may not be perceived by the child as wrong at first, because most victims know and trust their abusers.

  7. Munchausen syndrome by proxy is when a parent fabricates or causes symptoms in a child that results in the child being subjected to multiple invasive tests and treatments; the parent receives a great deal of attention from the health care team and is initially viewed as a very caring and attentive parent.

B. Assessment

  1. Do not examine the child alone; you could be implicated as the cause of the abuse.

  2. Observe parent-child interactions, carefully noting what the child and the parents say, including nonverbal communication.

  3. Describe each sore, bruise, or burn and its stage of healing.

  4. Note whether the injury or symptoms fit the history of the accident or illness.

  5. Note any delay in seeking help; ask the parents to explain why they did not seek immediate treatment.

  6. Suspect child abuse when a child's injury does not match the reported accident and when X-rays show old, unexplained fractures.

C. Interventions

  1. Meet the child's immediate physical and psychological needs first, regardless of suspicions.

  2. Protect the child; help the family begin to cope; try to prevent further abuse.

  3. Report suspected abuse to the proper authorities; this is mandated for nurses in all states.

  4. Reinforce what the parents do correctly; encourage their participation in the child's care.

  5. Teach the parents relevant child development principles; give them anticipatory guidance; serve as their role model.

  6. Provide consistent care to gain the parents' and child's trust.

  7. Engage the child in play that encourages the expression of feelings, especially guilt and fear.

  8. Refer the parents to a support group.

III. Attention-deficit/hyperactivity disorder (ADHD)

A. Overview
   1. The condition is thought to be due to a dysregulation of neurotransmitters, especially the catecholamines dopamine and norepinephrine in the prefrontal cortex.
   2. The prefrontal cortex is thought to be the site of executive behavior, such as decision making and attention.
   3. There is a genetic predisposition in 50% of cases.
   4. It does not usually affect one's ability to learn but rather affects the availability for learning to occur.

B. Assessment
   1. For the hyperactive impulsive type of ADHD:
      a) Fidgets with hands or feet/squirms in seat
      b) Leaves seat in situations when remaining seated is expected
      c) Runs/climbs excessively in situations in which it is inappropriate (adolescents have subjective feelings of restlessness)
      d) Has difficulty playing quietly
      e) Acts as if driven by a motor
      f) Talks excessively
      g) Blurts out answers before questions are completed
      h) Has difficulty awaiting turn
      i) Interrupts or intrudes on others
   2. For the inattentive type of ADHD:
      a) Fails to give close attention to details; makes careless mistakes
      b) Has difficulty sustaining attention in tasks
      c) Does not seem to listen when spoken to
      d) Does not follow through on instructions
      e) Has difficulty organizing tasks
      f) Avoids, reluctant to engage in tasks that require sustained mental effort
      g) Loses things necessary for tasks
      h) Easily distracted by extraneous stimuli
      i) Often forgetful in daily activities
   3. Child must have six of the nine criteria at a level significantly more than expected for age in a category to be diagnosed with that type.

4. Child must have the symptoms for >6 months.
5. Child must have the symptoms before age 7.
6. Symptoms must be present in at least two different settings (e.g., home and school).
7. Having at least six characteristics in both categories results in a diagnosis of combined ADHD.
8. Multiple psychiatric conditions are comorbid with ADHD; it is important to differentiate the symptoms of the various conditions.

C. Interventions
1. Psychostimulants are often prescribed to increase the availability of neurotransmitters to increase focus and attention.
   a) Most stimulant dosing is not weight dependent.
   b) Short-acting preparations last 4 hours; long-acting last 8 to 12 hours. Do not chew long-acting preparations as chewing destroys the delivery system.
   c) Common side effects include anorexia and sleep disturbances.
2. Implement behavioral/environmental interventions.
   a) Identify child's strengths and build on these.
   b) Have clear, simple rules.
   c) Develop a consistent routine in a structured but uncluttered environment.
   d) Get child's attention first before giving directions.
   e) Reduce environmental stimuli.

IV. Learning disabilities

A. Overview
1. Due to multiple causes, such as genetics, brain infections or trauma, cerebral radiation
2. Affects one's ability to process and use information by a particular modality thus affecting the ability to learn
3. Must have at least a normal IQ in order to have this diagnosis
4. Can be viewed from two frameworks:
   a) Reading, writing, or mathematical learning disabilities
   b) Sensory (visual and auditory), integrative, or motor learning disabilities

B. Assessment
   1. Visual perceptual sensory deficit
       a) Difficulty processing and/or interpreting information received visually; there is no vision deficit
       b) Dyslexia (reversing letters or words), difficulty copying or matching, difficulty differentiating a figure from the background, difficulty judging distance and speed, difficulty with visual memory
   2. Auditory perceptual sensory deficit
       a) Difficulty processing and/or interpreting information heard; there is no hearing deficit
       b) Difficulty reciting from memory, differentiating sounds, following oral directions, differentiating a sound from noise in the background
   3. Tactile perceptual sensory deficit
       a) Difficulty interpreting the sensations of the need to defecate or the start of menses
       b) May be hypersensitive to certain fabrics against the skin
   4. Integrative deficits
       a) Difficulty with sequencing information, problem solving, organizing, prioritizing
       b) Difficulty with abstract thought and with the concepts of science and mathematics
   5. Motor/expressive deficit
       a) Difficulty writing neatly, difficulty with hand-eye coordination

C. Interventions
   1. Teach child to compensate for the area of deficit.
   2. Use alternative modalities to teach child.
       a) If child has visual perceptual deficit, tape-record lesson and use hands-on learning.
       b) If child has auditory perceptual deficit, use checklists and use hands-on learning.
       c) If child has integrative deficit, use visual aids to sequence activities and pictures to describe amounts and the steps of a process.
       d) If child has motor deficits, use alternative modalities, such as computers, lined paper.
   3. Build self-esteem.

V. Autistic spectrum disorder

A. Overview
1. A pervasive developmental disorder that includes a spectrum of conditions, including autism, Rett syndrome, and Asperger's syndrome
2. Is of unknown cause
3. Must be present from birth
4. Must be differentiated from mental retardation, deafness, and childhood schizophrenia
5. Characterized by severe and pervasive impairment in reciprocal social interaction and communication skills, as well as restricted and repetitive behaviors

B. Assessment
1. Note that the child does not relate to or interact with others.
2. Observe that the child does not cuddle or mold to the body of the caretaker.
3. Note that the child does not demonstrate anticipatory behaviors as the parent approaches.
4. Note that the child does not appear to be comforted by the parent's touch after an injury.
5. Observe that the child uses peripheral vision rather than central vision; the child looks past you and avoids eye contact.
6. The child may not have meaningful speech.
   a) Uses inappropriate noises and responses
   b) Appears deaf, but is not
7. Note that if speech is present, the child rarely refers to self and uses echolalia, where the child repeats what he/she hears over and over.
8. The child appears fascinated by objects that spin, reflect light, sparkle, or are smooth; child prefers inanimate objects but may relate to pets.
9. The child performs repetitive motions and self-stimulating behaviors, such as rocking; the child appears hyperactive.
10. Note that the child does not appear to be anxious when separated from parents.
11. The child demonstrates inappropriate fears of harmless items.
12. The child resists a change in routines.

C. Interventions
1. Work with the child on a one-to-one relationship.
2. Give the child specific directions to follow, initially without rationales.
3. Minimize handling to prevent upsetting the child.
4. Decrease stimulation in the environment.
5. Initiate a goal of getting the child to be aware of others.
6. Provide the family with support.

VI. Eating disorders: Anorexia and bulimia

A. Overview
1. Common in adolescents
2. Often the result of poor perception of the physical self or poor self-esteem

B. Anorexia nervosa
1. A voluntary refusal to eat accompanied by weighing less than 85% of the expected normal weight without an organic cause and intense fear of gaining weight and becoming fat
2. Results from a distorted, unrealistic attitude toward body size, body weight, and intake that overrides feelings of hunger, threats by family, or accurate knowledge

C. Bulimia (binge-purge)
1. A ravenous appetite and huge intake followed by feelings of guilt and anxiety and resulting in forced vomiting; these are referred to as binge-purge cycles

D. Assessment
1. Measure height, weight, and muscle mass.
2. Assess for metabolic alkalosis from vomiting.
3. Note electrolyte status, especially potassium; assess cardiac function.
4. Note signs of malnutrition, such as amenorrhea, mood changes, intentional periods of overactivity, loss of libido, and bradycardia.
5. Has the previously pubertal teen ceased having menstrual periods?
6. Does the youth use enemas, laxatives, diuretics, or diet pills?
7. Induced vomiting may cause sore throat, dental decay, and irritated fingers.
8. Assess for cold intolerance, dry skin, hair loss, orthostatic hypotension.
9. Assess intake and output.

E. Interventions
   1. Recommend psychotherapy.
   2. Behavior modification may be helpful to decrease the adolescent's manipulative behavior.
   3. Institute measures to remove anger and anxiety from the eating situation.
   4. Work with the adolescent to plan well-balanced meals with adequate caloric intake.
   5. Be a role model.

VII. Anxiety disorders

A. Overview
   1. Common among children of all ages
   2. Includes separation anxiety, generalized anxiety, panic disorders, phobias, posttraumatic stress disorder, and obsessive-compulsive disorder

B. Assessment
   1. Assess vital signs for tachycardia and tachypnea; the child may complain of shortness of breath.
   2. Assess for diaphoresis, tremors, nausea, stomachache, and headache.
   3. Ask about sleep problems and nightmares.
   4. Assess for decreased participation in normal activities.
   5. Assess for self-esteem.
   6. Ask about school performance.
   7. Ask if the teen has used drugs or alcohol to dull the sensations.

C. Interventions
   1. Initiate relaxation exercises.
      a) Encourage diaphragmatic breathing (breathe in through the nose and out through the mouth).
   2. Promote participation in professional counseling.
   3. Promote self-esteem.

VIII. Mood disorders

A. Overview
   1. Includes depression, bipolar disorder, and suicidal ideation.
   2. Sadness lasts longer than is common in children and interferes with social functioning, concentration on academic work, and feelings about self.

  B. Assessment

    1. Be aware that psychosomatic complaints may be a "call for help."

    2. Ask questions such as, "What makes you sad?" "What are some things you worry about?" "What do you do when you feel sad?"

    3. Assess for self-mutilation, such as cutting, and self-destructive behaviors, such as the use of drugs and alcohol.

  C. Interventions

    1. Professional therapy is usually needed.

    2. Selective serotonin reuptake inhibitors (SSRI) may be prescribed.

IX. Suicide ideation

  A. Overview

    1. Third leading cause of death among adolescents

  B. Assessment

    1. Has the youth made comments about being better off if dead?

    2. Does the youth have thoughts about killing himself or herself?

    3. Does the youth have a plan to kill himself or herself?

    4. Does the youth have a weapon to kill himself or herself?

    5. Has the youth engaged in cutting of or abusing his or her skin?

  C. Intervention

    1. Stay with the child; do not leave the child alone.

    2. Contact parents or psychiatrist and stay with child until resource people arrive.

CHAPTER
18

Issues and the Law

LEARNING OBJECTIVES

1. Describe the rights guaranteed to children by IDEA and Section 504 of the Rehabilitation Act

2. Define an Emancipated Minor

I. Individuals with Disabilities Education Improvement Act (IDEA)

A. Guarantees that children with disabilities will receive a "free and appropriate public education in the least restrictive environment"

B. Guarantees that children thought to have disabilities will be evaluated free of charge

C. Guarantees that an Individualized Education Program (IEP) be developed by a team of specialists and include the parents. This will identify the special education and related services that will be provided for the child.

D. Requires that a transition plan be developed by age 16 to assist the student to plan for transition to vocational training, postsecondary education, or assisted living/complete care facilities

   1. Nurses should be assisting patients to begin planning to make the transition from pediatric care to adult care.

E. Requires early intervention identification of infants and toddlers with disabilities and initiation of measures that will assist the child to enter school in a state of readiness

   1. Requires the development of an Individualized Family Service Plan to identify the needed services and to coordinate the plan of care

II. Section 504 of the Rehabilitation Act of 1973

A. Civil rights law that prohibits discrimination on the basis of disability in programs that receive federal financial assistance

B. States that no qualified individual with a disability shall be excluded from, denied the benefits of, or subjected to discrimination under any program that receives financial assistance

C. Requires that reasonable accommodations be made to assist the individual in being successful. This may require wider doors for wheelchairs; ramps/curb cuts/elevators for those in wheelchairs; special desks and chairs; computers, telecommunication devices, or special devices for communication; performing tube feedings or percussion and postural drainage within the school setting so that the child can attend school.

D. The development of a 504 plan details the accommodations needed by the individual.

III. Health Insurance Portability and Accountability Act (HIPAA)

A. HIPAA protects the privacy of patients' medical records and other identifiable health information.

B. Patients can obtain copies of their medical records and request changes if they identify errors.

C. Personal health information generally may not be used for purposes not related to health care.

D. Assure confidentiality when communicating health-related information about a patient.

IV. Emancipated minor

A. The granting of basic adult rights; definition varies among states and not all states recognize emancipated minor status

B. Generally includes the following:
1. Under age 18 and usually older than age 14
2. Legally married
3. On active military duty
4. Minors who can demonstrate maturity and financial independence; may have to make a legal informed declaration

C. Parents no longer required to pay financial support

D. Assume responsibility for their own medical coverage

E. Give consent for all medical care, without parental consent, knowledge, or liability

F. Can enter into a binding contract; can consent to participate in research

Practice Test

181 Questions

Chapter 1:
Introduction to Pediatric Nursing Certification Review

No questions

Chapter 2:
Overview of Pediatric Nursing

1. A 2-year-old who is chronically ill is being admitted to the inpatient unit for pain control. Her mother tells you that she feels guilty leaving her in the hospital because she cries so much. As the nurse caring for this child, the most appropriate explanation to the mother would be

   a. The child will stop crying as soon as you leave.
   b. Crying is a sign of attachment, but you need time for yourself too.
   c. It's always hard to leave your child, but once you do you will feel much better.
   d. She is crying because she is uncomfortable, not because you are leaving.

2. A mother of a 3½-year-old cannot stay in the hospital with her child today. The nurse suggests the mother do which of the following:

   a. The mother visit at the same time daily for the same amount of time.
   b. The mother explain that she'll be right back.
   c. The mother leave while the child is distracted or sleeping.
   d. The mother leave one of her possessions behind for the child.

Answer Key

1. b
2. d

Chapter 3:
Growth and Development

1. **The principles of growth and development include all of the following except**

    a. Each child grows and develops according to a general orderly pattern that tends to resemble that of others of the same age, sex, and nationality.
    b. Development proceeds in a cephalocaudal and proximodistal manner.
    c. Development proceeds from the specific to the general.
    d. Growth and development are interrelated and interdependent.

2. **The period of greatest growth is from**

    a. Birth to 1 year
    b. Toddlerhood to preschool years
    c. School age to preadolescence
    d. The beginning to the end of adolescence

3. **A developmentally appropriate 3½-year-old child is likely to be most fearful of which of the following activities?**

    a. Chest X-ray
    b. Rectal temperature
    c. Bed bath by the nurse
    d. Blood pressure

4. **The neonatal period begins at birth and lasts for 4 weeks. During this time, the infant adapts to the extrauterine environment. Which of the following is true about the neonate?**

    a. The sense of hearing is immature.
    b. Myelinization of the brain is complete.
    c. The anterior fontanel will close within a month.
    d. Temperature-regulating mechanisms are immature.

5. **Four-year-old Juan is being admitted today for a tonsillectomy. You know that Juan is in which developmental stage according to Erikson?**

   a. Initiative versus guilt
   b. Identity versus role confusion
   c. Industry versus inferiority
   d. Autonomy versus shame and doubt

6. **Which of the following criteria is used in assessing readiness for toilet training?**

   a. The child should be at least 2 years old before toilet training.
   b. The child can demonstrate an awareness that she is urinating and defecating.
   c. The child should have a dry diaper through the night.
   d. The child should have resolved her fears about what might happen when she flushes the toilet.

7. **Thomas is a 6-month-old who weighed 6 lb at birth. Based on your knowledge of pediatric growth, you know that his weight today should be at least**

   a. 9 lb
   b. 12 lb
   c. 16 lb
   d. 18 lb

8. **You are preparing to measure the length of 12-month-old William. His mother tells you he was 20 inches at birth. Based on your knowledge of normal growth parameters you would expect his length to be approximately**

   a. 25% greater than his birth length
   b. 50% greater than his birth length
   c. 75% greater than his birth length
   d. Double his birth length

9. **Dana is a 30-month-old female whose length you are plotting. You measured her using a length board. Which growth chart would you choose?**

    a. Girls: 0-36 months
    b. Girls: 2-18 years
    c. Either a girls 0-36 months or a 2-18 years growth chart; it does not matter
    d. You must plot on both charts since she's in the transitional period

10. **When performing a well-child assessment of a 4-month-old, which of the following represents a normal assessment finding?**

    a. Closed anterior and posterior fontanel
    b. Open anterior and posterior fontanel
    c. Closed anterior and open posterior fontanel
    d. Open anterior and closed posterior fontanel

11. **A bottle-fed infant, age 3 months, is brought to the pediatrician's office for a well-child visit. During the previous visit, the nurse taught the mother about infant nutritional needs. Which statement by the mother during the current visit indicates effective teaching?**

    a. "I started the baby on cereals and fruits because he wasn't sleeping through the night."
    b. "I started putting cereal in the bottle with formula because the baby kept spitting it out when I gave it with a spoon."
    c. "I'm giving the baby iron-fortified formula and a fluoride supplement because our water isn't fluoridated."
    d. "I'm giving the baby skim milk because he was getting so chubby."

12. **When assessing the development of a 3-month-old, which of the following would be most concerning?**

    a. Failure to look for objects when they are no longer in the visual field
    b. Failure to smile
    c. Failure to roll over
    d. Failure to pull feet to mouth

13. **When assessing the 7-month-old, which of the following is he most likely to be developing?**

    a. Rocking back and forth on hands and knees
    b. Standing while holding onto an object for support
    c. Waving bye-bye
    d. Rolling over

14. **Which of the following is *not* well developed in a newborn infant?**

    a. Hearing
    b. Vision
    c. Touch
    d. Pain sensation

15. **Introduction of a cup to drink fluids can begin as early as what age?**

    a. 3 months
    b. 6 months
    c. 9 months
    d. 12 months

16. **You are educating the mother of an infant about growth and nutrition. You know that the earliest age at which the infant should be changed from formula or breast milk to whole milk is**

    a. 6 months
    b. 9 months
    c. 12 months
    d. 15 months

17. **You are the nurse in a community heath center and are responsible for reviewing anticipatory guidance and safety education with parents who bring young children for health assessments. You are educating the parents of 12-month-old Alyssa who weighs 18 pounds. Which of the following is the most accurate anticipatory guidance for Alyssa's parents regarding car seat installation? Alyssa should sit in a**

    a. Forward-facing car seat in the rear of the automobile
    b. Forward-facing car seat in the passenger seat of the automobile
    c. Rear-facing car seat in the rear of the automobile
    d. Rear-facing car safety seat in the passenger seat of the automobile

18. **Which of the following types of play would the nurse expect to see when assessing a toddler?**

    a. Cooperative
    b. Associative
    c. Solitary
    d. Parallel

19. **Four-year-old Rebecca, who is hospitalized for treatment of a brain tumor, tells her nurse that she got sick because she was a bad girl. Which of the following would the nurse identify as the underlying rationale for this statement?**

    a. Magical thinking
    b. Egocentrism
    c. Self-blame
    d. Conservation

20. **A 4-year-old who is blind is hospitalized. You bring in her dinner tray. How do you tell her where her food is?**

    a. Set the food up like a clock.
    b. Tell her which food is on the left and right.
    c. Tell her you will feed her to make it easier for her to eat.
    d. Place one food at a time in front of her.

21. **A mother brings her 10-month-old son to the pediatrician's office. When the nurse approaches to measure the child's vital signs, he clings to his mother tightly and starts to cry. The mother says, "He used to smile at everyone. I don't know why he's acting this way." Which response by the nurse would help the mother understand her child's behavior?**

    a. "Your baby's behavior indicates stranger anxiety, which is common at his age."
    b. "Children who behave that way are developing shy personalities."
    c. "Children at this age begin to fear pain."
    d. "Your baby's having a temper tantrum, which is common at his age."

22. **A child, age 5, is brought to the pediatrician's office for a routine visit. When inspecting the child's mouth, the nurse expects to find how many teeth?**

    a. Up to 10
    b. Up to 15
    c. Up to 20
    d. Up to 32

23. **When telling a 4-year-old child about an upcoming procedure, the nurse's most important consideration is to**

    a. Tell the child immediately before the procedure is to occur.
    b. Prepare the child at least 24 hours in advance so that the child has time to emotionally adjust.
    c. Offer a toy to keep the child happy and distracted.
    d. Wait to tell the child until you are doing the procedure.

24. **An 18-month-old child, immobilized with traction to the legs, has a nursing diagnosis of diversional activity deficit related to immobility. The nurse should include playing with which diversional activity in the plan of care?**

    a. Tinkertoys
    b. A pounding board
    c. A pull toy
    d. Board games

25. **A parent calls the clinic to express concern over her child's eating habits. She says the child eats very little and consumes only a single type of food for weeks on end. The nurse knows that this behavior is characteristic of children ages**

    a. 2-4 years
    b. 5-8 years
    c. 9-12 years
    d. 13-17 years

26. When assessing a toddler's growth and development, the nurse understands that a child in this age group displays behavior that fosters which developmental task?

    a. Initiative
    b. Autonomy
    c. Trust
    d. Industry

27. The nurse should expect a 3-year-old child to be able to perform which action?

    a. Roller-skate
    b. Tie shoe laces
    c. Ride a tricycle
    d. Jump rope

28. When performing a physical assessment on a girl, age 10, the nurse keeps in mind that the first sign of sexual maturity in girls is

    a. Axillary hair
    b. Pubic hair
    c. Breast bud development
    d. Menarche

29. When developing a plan of care for an adolescent, the nurse considers the child's psychosocial needs. During adolescence, psychosocial development focuses on

    a. Becoming industrious
    b. Establishing an identity
    c. Achieving intimacy
    d. Developing initiative

30. An 9-month-old infant is hospitalized for treatment of inorganic failure to thrive. Which nursing action is most appropriate for this child?

    a. Encouraging the infant to hold his bottle
    b. Keeping the infant on bed rest to conserve energy
    c. Rotating caregivers to provide more stimulation
    d. Maintaining a consistent, structured environment

31. **The nurse suspects that a child, age 4, is being neglected physically. To best assess the child's nutritional status, the nurse should start by asking the parents which of the following questions?**

    a. "Has your child always been so thin?"
    b. "Is your child a picky eater?"
    c. "What did your child eat for breakfast today?"
    d. "Do you have difficulty buying nutritious foods at the supermarket?

32. **A child, age 15 months, is recovering from surgery to remove a Wilms' tumor. Which finding best indicates that the child is experiencing pain, even though the child is denying it?**

    a. Increased appetite
    b. Increased heart rate
    c. Decreased urine output
    d. Increased interest in television

33. **A school-age child with a chronic condition is hospitalized for the fourth time this year. What would be most appropriate strategy related to contact with the school?**

    a. Have her mother go to the school to get her missed homework.
    b. Have the school nurse come to visit.
    c. Make arrangements for the child to be homeschooled so that she does not fall behind in her studies.
    d. Have her classmates send her letters wishing her a good recovery.

Answer Key

1. c	12. b	23. a
2. a	13. a	24. b
3. b	14. b	25. a
4. d	15. b	26. b
5. a	16. c	27. c
6. b	17. c	28. c
7. b	18. d	29. b
8. b	19. a	30. d
9. a	20. d	31. c
10. d	21. a	32. b
11. c	22. c	33. d

Chapter 4:
Genetic Alterations

1. Justin is an 8-year-old with cystic fibrosis. His mother wants to conceive again. What genetic counseling can you give regarding her chances of having another child with the disease for her next pregnancy?

    a.   100%
    b.   75%
    c.   50%
    d.   25%

2. Parents of a child with hemophilia ask you what are the chances of having another child with hemophilia. You correctly tell them:

    a.   25% of your children; all will be carriers
    b.   50% of your sons; none of your daughters
    c.   100% of your sons; 50% of your daughters
    d.   25% of your sons; none of your daughters

Answer Key
1. d
2. b

Chapter 5:
Hematologic Conditions

1. **Which of the following is not a risk factor for iron deficiency anemia?**

    a. Being part of a multiple birth
    b. Being premature
    c. Being an adolescent
    d. Being school age

2. **Which of the following children would be at greatest risk for anemia?**

    a. Infant with asthma
    b. Toddler with Down syndrome
    c. School-age child with nephrotic syndrome
    d. Adolescent with pelvic inflammatory disease

3. **You are instructing the mother of an infant with iron deficiency anemia about the administration of iron. Which of the following is the most accurate information to teach the mother about when to give the iron supplement?**

    a. 15 minutes before meals to improve absorption
    b. With meals and with milk to improve absorption
    c. Between meals and with orange juice to improve absorption
    d. Within 15 minutes after eating a meal to decrease GI distress

4. **The lifespan of the normal red blood cell is**

    a. 120 days
    b. 90 days
    c. 45 days
    d. 10 days

5. **Five-year-old Sam was admitted today to the unit for complications of hereditary spherocytosis. You would expect to see all of the following symptoms except:**

    a. Splenomegaly
    b. A low hemoglobin count
    c. Jaundice
    d. A decreased reticulocyte count

6. The mother of a 6-month-old child with sickle cell disease asks you why the infant has not had any symptoms prior to this time. You explain to her that many young infants with sickle cell disease do not have symptoms of the disease because they have high levels of:

   a. Maternal antibodies
   b. Hemoglobin S
   c. Hemoglobin F
   d. Hemoglobin A

7. A 6-year-old child with sickle cell disease is being admitted to the inpatient unit today with vaso-occlusive crisis. Your priority nursing intervention will be which of the following?

   a. Administering antibiotics
   b. Promoting hydration and oxygenation
   c. Assessing spleen size and protecting it from trauma
   d. Restricting fluids and assessing for edema

8. You are caring for a neonate admitted to the unit for treatment of hyperbilirubinemia. Which of the following would *not* be part of the nursing care for the child receiving phototherapy?

   a. Assess hydration status and stooling pattern.
   b. Assure eye shields are in place.
   c. Monitor neurologic status.
   d. Provide a light t-shirt to maintain thermoregulation.

9. Aaron is a 2-year-old with severe hemophilia (factor VIII deficiency) who was hospitalized today for hemarthrosis of the knee. As the nurse caring for him, your nursing priorities include which of the following?

   a. Encourage active range of motion while in bed.
   b. Discuss use of a helmet at home.
   c. Teach the parent how to administer factor VIII at home.
   d. Keep the knee immobilized and elevated above the heart.

10. David is a 10-year-old recently diagnosed with ITP. He is an active boy who is a member of his school basketball team. You are the nurse discharging David from the hospital. David's platelet count is 19,000 with some petechiae, but no serious bleeding at present. Which of the following would be most important to include in the discharge teaching for David and his parents?

    a. Immediately discontinue participation in his school basketball team.

    b. Encourage aspirin instead of acetaminophen for pain.

    c. Provide information about a splenectomy that may occur in the near future.

    d. Massage the skin daily to increase circulation.

11. For the child with hemophilia, what is the most important nursing goal?

    a. Enhancing tissue perfusion

    b. Preventing bleeding episodes

    c. Promoting tissue oxygenation

    d. Controlling pain

12. A toddler with hemophilia is hospitalized with multiple injuries after falling off a sliding board. X-rays reveal no bone fractures. When caring for the child, what is the nurse's highest priority?

    a. Administering platelets, as prescribed

    b. Taking measures to prevent infection

    c. Frequently assessing the child's level of consciousness

    d. Discussing a safe play environment with the parents

Answer Key

1.	d	5.	d	9.	d
2.	c	6.	c	10.	a
3.	c	7.	b	11.	b
4.	a	8.	d	12.	c

Chapter 6:
Infectious Diseases

1. The *Haemophilus influenzae* vaccine has contributed to a decreased incidence in which of the following conditions among children?

    a. Measles
    b. Chickenpox
    c. Epiglottitis
    d. Polio

2. Which method of immune protection has the highest level of side effects?

    a. Naturally acquired active
    b. Naturally acquired passive
    c. Artificially acquired active
    d. Artificially acquired passive

3. Which of the following is the best location for administration of an intramuscular injection in an infant or toddler?

    a. Dorsogluteal muscle
    b. Deltoid muscle
    c. Buttocks
    d. Vastus lateralis muscle

4. A toddler has been admitted to the unit for treatment of measles. You would expect to see each of the following *except*?

    a. Koplik's spots
    b. Photophobia
    c. Swelling of the parotid glands and painful swallowing
    d. A maculopapular, red, pruritic rash

5. **You are the community health nurse performing well-child assessments at the local community health center. Mrs. Rodriguez returns to the clinic to report a positive PPD result for her 15-month-old daughter Rose. Which of the following statements is the most appropriate response to Mrs. Rodriguez?**

   a. "It is common to have a false-positive result on the PPD test, so the first thing we should do is another PPD."

   b. "Rose has active tuberculosis. She needs to begin wearing a mask immediately."

   c. "Rose has active tuberculosis but is likely not contagious. She should start antibiotics today."

   d. "Rose has been exposed to tuberculosis. She will need to get a chest X- ray as soon as possible to determine if her lungs show signs of tuberculosis disease."

6. **Which of the following would be the most appropriate anticipatory guidance statement for the nurse to give regarding a 12-year-old male with mononucleosis?**

   a. He should stay home from school for at least 48 hours until the antibiotics have taken effect.

   b. He should avoid contact sports because of the risk of splenic rupture.

   c. It is important that he take the full dose of antibiotics.

   d. He should resume all activities as soon as he regains his energy.

7. **You are the telephone triage nurse at the local pediatric primary care health center. Mrs. Hall calls you to ask when she can expect her son Johnny to be able to return to school. He broke out with chickenpox 2 days ago. The best anticipatory guidance for Mrs. Hall is**

   a. "It is impossible to determine when he can return to school. We'll just wait and see."

   b. "His skin must be completely clear. This takes approximately 2 weeks."

   c. "Johnny can return to school once all of the chickenpox are scabbed over."

   d. "Once the chickenpox erupt, children are no longer contagious. Once Johnny's fever resolves and he is feeling better he may return to school."

8. **Emma is 9 months old. You would expect that she should have received how many of which immunizations at this age?**

    a. 2 Hepatitis, 3 DTaP, 2 Hib, and 2 IPV
    b. 3 DTaP, 3 doses of oral polio vaccine, and 2 Hib
    c. 4 DTaP, 1 MMR, 1 varicella, and 1 Hib
    d. 3 DTaP, 1 MMR, 2 Hib, and 3 IPV

9. **When teaching parents about fifth disease (erythema infectiosum) and its transmission, the nurse should provide information that the disease is transmitted by**

    a. Respiratory secretions
    b. An unknown mode of transmission
    c. Blood and body secretions
    d. Stool and hand-to-mouth contamination

10. **Heather is 12 months old and comes to the pediatric clinic for a checkup. She has not been to the clinic since she was 2 months old, at which point she received a DTaP and hepatitis vaccine. Because it has been 10 months since her last vaccination, you know that today she should receive which immunizations?**

    a. Start over with the immunizations, since it has been too long since the first shots. Give DTaP, Hib, and IPV.
    b. She should receive the second dose of each immunization. Give DTaP and hepatitis vaccine.
    c. Give all vaccines appropriate for a 12-month-old. Give DTaP, hepatitis B, Hib, IPV, MMR, and varicella.
    d. Because of her age, only give the MMR and varicella and instruct the parent to bring her back every month to update the rest of her immunizations.

Answer Key

1.	c	6.	b
2.	a	7.	c
3.	d	8.	a
4.	c	9.	a
5.	d	10.	c

Chapter 7:
Immune System Dysfunction

1. An infant born to an HIV-positive mother should receive which of the following drug categories shortly after birth?

    a. Corticosteroids, such as prednisone
    b. β2-Agonists, such as albuterol
    c. Antivirals, such as zidovudine
    d. Antibiotics, such as erythromycin

2. Which of the following would be the most important part of prevention teaching for the mother of an 8-month-old with eczema?

    a. Avoid nylon clothing.
    b. Bathe only two or three times per week and avoid soap.
    c. The child should begin allergy shots as soon as the allergen is identified.
    d. Apply emollient creams liberally after daily baths.

3. Sally is a 4-year-old with type I respiratory allergies. With what preventive measures will you instruct the parent to assist Sally?

    a. Use dry dusting to prevent the growth of mold.
    b. Keep the house carpeted to provide warmth and safety.
    c. Use only natural fibers, such as down pillows and wool fabrics.
    d. Keep Sally indoors with the windows closed when the grass is being cut.

4. Which of the following laboratory values would give the most helpful information about a child's ability to fight infection?

    a. White blood cell count
    b. Absolute neutrophil count
    c. Sedimentation rate
    d. Red blood cell count

5. **Which of the following interventions would you recommend the parent give to a healthy child with a fever of 102.5 °F?**

    a.   A cool-water bath
    b.   An alcohol bath
    c.   Aspirin
    d.   Acetaminophen

6. **A 14-month-old child with acquired immunodeficiency syndrome (AIDS) is admitted to the hospital with an infection. When developing a plan of care, the nurse must keep in mind that AIDS in children is commonly is associated with**

    a.   Kaposi's sarcoma
    b.   Congenital heart anomalies
    c.   Developmental delays
    d.   Bleeding disorders

7. **A woman who has tested positive for the human immunodeficiency virus (HIV) delivers a girl. When she asks if her baby has AIDS, how should the nurse respond?**

    a.   "Don't worry. It's too soon to tell."
    b.   "Chances are she'll be okay because you don't have AIDS yet."
    c.   "She may have acquired HIV in utero, but we won't know for sure for a few months."
    d.   "Almost all babies born to HIV-positive women are infected with HIV. But your baby won't have symptoms for years."

8. **Katlyn had myelomeningocele repair at birth. She requires catheterization multiple times each day. Now, at age 8, she has developed an allergy to latex. Which of the following statements will guide your nursing interventions when Katlyn is hospitalized?**

    a.   Latex allergies can occur both by contact and by inhalation of latex particles.
    b.   Because latex is in rubber gloves, do not use gloves during the catheterization procedure.
    c.   Hospitals are now, by law, latex-free, so no additional measures need to be taken.
    d.   Katlyn should be in protective isolation to prevent contact with any latex.

Answer Key

1.	c	5.	d
2.	b	6.	c
3.	d	7.	c
4.	b	8.	a

Chapter 8:

Cancer

1. **You are the nurse caring for 9-year-old Bethany, who has acute lymphoblastic leukemia and is unconscious and close to death. Your most appropriate action is to**

    a. Remain with Bethany and her parents as much as possible.
    b. Spend the usual amount of time with Bethany in her room.
    c. Allow Bethany and her parents to have as much time as possible to be together alone.
    d. Encourage the parents to go home so they don't have to watch her die.

2. **Which of the following is true about acute lymphoblastic leukemia?**

    a. It is the most common type of childhood cancer in adolescents.
    b. Its prognosis for a 5-year survival is less than 50%.
    c. It is associated with increased blast cells in the bone marrow.
    d. It has a high genetic predisposition.

3. **Which of the following is most likely to be seen in the child with leukemia?**

    a. Night sweats and lymphadenopathy
    b. Abdominal distention
    c. History of fractures
    d. Bruising and fatigue

4. **Amanda is a toddler who has been diagnosed with Wilms' tumor. A priority nursing intervention is the avoidance of what?**

    a. Foods high in carbohydrates
    b. Palpation of the abdomen
    c. Latex products
    d. Intramuscular injections

5. **The primary pathophysiology of acute lymphoblastic leukemia is due to**

    a. Excessive destruction of red blood cells by hemolysis
    b. Excessive exposure to radiation
    c. Deficient production of mature blood cells by the bone marrow
    d. Inability of the liver to make the necessary clotting factors

6. **Joseph is a preschooler who is being evaluated for a potential diagnosis of leukemia. The mother asks you how the diagnosis is made. You know that the definitive test for a diagnosis of leukemia is**

    a. Bone marrow aspiration
    b. Complete white blood cell count and differential
    c. Lumbar puncture
    d. Clotting time/prothrombin time

7. **Jill's platelet count is 10,000. As her nurse, your priority is to observe for which of the following?**

    a. Excessive bleeding
    b. Signs of anemia
    c. Cardiac failure
    d. Signs of infection

8. **Which is a priority nursing measure for the child receiving radiation therapy for cancer?**

    a. Restrict fluids to decrease nausea.
    b. Do not remove the skin markings for the radiation fields.
    c. Culture all orifices four times each day.
    d. Place in isolation for droplet precautions.

9. **A child, age 5, has acute lymphoblastic leukemia and is to receive induction chemotherapy consisting of vincristine, asparaginase, and prednisone. When teaching the parents about the adverse effects of this regimen, the nurse should stress the importance of promptly reporting**

    a. Hair loss
    b. Moon face
    c. Constipation
    d. Bone pain

10. **A child experiences nausea and vomiting after receiving cancer chemotherapy drugs. To help prevent these problems from recurring, the nurse should**

    a. Provide a high-fiber diet before the next chemotherapy session

    b. Administer allopurinol 2 hours before the next chemotherapy session

    c. Encourage increased fluid intake before the next chemotherapy session

    d. Administer an antiemetic 30 to 60 minutes before the next chemotherapy session

11. **A child, age 4, is diagnosed with leukemia. She complains of being tired and sleeps most of the day. Which nursing diagnosis reflects the nurse's understanding of the physiologic effects of leukemia?**

    a. Ineffective airway clearance related to fatigue

    b. Activity intolerance related to anemia

    c. Altered nutrition: more than body requirements related to lack of activity

    d. Impaired tissue perfusion related to central nervous system infiltration by leukemic cells

12. **A child, age 15 months, is admitted to the hospital. During the initial nursing assessment, which statement by the mother will be most helpful in assessing for Wilms' tumor?**

    a. "My child has grown 3 inches in the past 6 months."

    b. "My child seems to be napping for longer periods."

    c. "My child's abdomen seems bigger, and the diapers are much tighter."

    d. My child's appetite has increased so much lately."

13. **A 16-year-old adolescent has just been diagnosed with osteogenic sarcoma. What sign might have helped to make this diagnosis?**

    a. Pathologic fractures

    b. Petechiae

    c. Splenomegaly

    d. Headaches that are more common in the morning on rising

14. A school-age child is admitted to the hospital with a diagnosis of acute lymphoblastic leukemia. The nurse formulates a nursing diagnosis of risk for infection. What is the most effective way for the nurse to reduce the child's risk for infection?

    a. Restrict visitors to the patient to only the parents.
    b. Maintain universal precautions.
    c. Require staff and visitors to wear masks.
    d. Practice thorough hand washing.

15. The parents of a 4-year-old child in the terminal phase of a fatal illness ask the nurse for guidance in discussing death with their child. Which response is appropriate?

    a. "Children of that age view death as temporary and reversible, which makes it hard to explain."
    b. "Children of that age typically fantasize about what dying will be like, which is much better than knowing the truth."
    c. "At this developmental stage, children are afraid of death, so it's best not to discuss it with them."
    d. "At this developmental stage, most children have an adult concept of death and should be encouraged to discuss it."

Answer Key

1. a	6. a	11. b
2. c	7. a	12. c
3. d	8. b	13. a
4. b	9. d	14. d
5. c	10. d	15. a

Chapter 9:
Cardiac Conditions

1. **You are the nurse in the inpatient cardiac unit caring for a 10-year-old child receiving digoxin. Which of the following would be a priority assessment?**

    a. Apical pulse prior to administration
    b. Blood pressure prior to administration
    c. Temperature prior to administration
    d. Ensure adequate hydration prior to administration

2. **Five-year-old Sarah was admitted for cardiac surgery. She has tetralogy of Fallot. In comparing Sarah with a healthy 5-year-old girl, the differences you would expect to see in Sarah's growth are**

    a. Shorter in stature, heavier in weight, delayed dentition
    b. Average stature, lighter in weight, delayed dentition
    c. Taller in stature, delayed dentition, and muscles more firm
    d. Shorter in stature, lighter in weight, muscles less firm

3. **The abnormal changes in heart structure in tetralogy of Fallot are**

    a. Stenosis of the pulmonary vein, hypertrophy of the right ventricle, dextroposition of the aorta, and an ventricular septal defect
    b. Hypertrophy of the left ventricle, stenosis of the pulmonary vein, atrial septal defect, and dextroposition of the aorta.
    c. Stenosis of the pulmonary artery, hypertrophy of the right ventricle, ventricular septal defect, and dextroposition of the aorta
    d. Stenosis of the pulmonary artery, hypertrophy of the left ventricle, a patent ductus arteriosus, and dextroposition of the aorta

4. When a child is diagnosed with coarctation of the aorta, why is the surgery scheduled in early childhood instead of waiting until an older age?

    a. To increase the electrolytes circulating in the lower half of the body
    b. To avoid the effects of prolonged hypertension
    c. To prevent liver failure
    d. To increase the pedal pulse pressure

5. Which of the following is an important well-child assessment to evaluate for undiagnosed coarctation of the aorta in children?

    a. Cardiac assessment for murmurs
    b. Hematologic monitoring of hemoglobin
    c. Assessment of exercise tolerance
    d. Assessment of four extremity blood pressures

6. A 10-month-old infant with tetralogy of Fallot experiences a cyanotic episode, or "tet spell." To improve oxygenation during an episode, the nurse should place the infant in which position?

    a. Knee-to-chest
    b. Fowler's
    c. Trendelenburg
    d. Prone

7. A 4-year-old with a cyanotic heart condition is observed squatting on the floor next to her bed playing with a stuffed animal. Your first action is which of the following?

    a. Pick her up and place her in bed with an oxygen mask.
    b. As long as she appears comfortable, take no action, but observe her.
    c. Encourage her to stand and walk around the room to enhance circulation.
    d. Contact the physician.

8. **Laboratory results for a child with cyanotic congenital heart defect reveal an elevated hemoglobin level, hematocrit, and red blood cell count. What do these data suggest?**

    a. Anemia
    b. Dehydration
    c. Jaundice
    d. Compensation for hypoxia

9. **A child, age 3, is hospitalized for treatment of Kawasaki disease. During the acute phase of this disease, the nurse must assess the child for**

    a. Level of consciousness
    b. Kidney failure
    c. Desquamation of the hands and feet
    d. Hepatitis

10. **A child with suspected rheumatic fever is admitted to the pediatric unit. When obtaining the child's history, the nurse considers which information to be most important?**

    a. A fever that started 3 days ago
    b. Lack of interest in food
    c. A recent episode of pharyngitis
    d. Vomiting for 2 days

11. **What is your best explanation to a 12-year-old who has just asked you to explain why he has rheumatic fever?**

    a. "Your immune system has mistaken your heart valves as bacteria and is attacking your own heart."
    b. "You have an infection in your heart."
    c. "Your heart is having trouble handling an infection that is in your bloodstream."
    d. "This is a condition that can easily be treated with antibiotics."

12. **Which assessment finding is an early sign of congestive heart failure in a toddler?**

      a.   Increased respiratory rate
      b.   Increased urine output
      c.   Decreased weight
      d.   Decreased heart rate

Answer Key

1.	a		7.	b
2.	d		8.	d
3.	c		9.	c
4.	b		10.	c
5.	d		11.	a
6.	a		12.	a

Chapter 10:

Respiratory Conditions

1. **What is the most appropriate equipment to have available for the child arriving in the emergency department with suspected epiglottitis?**

    a. Bag-mask and bronchodilators
    b. Tracheostomy setup and oxygen
    c. Suction setup and oxygen
    d. Antibiotics and suction

2. **You are the nurse caring for a 16-year-old female with cystic fibrosis. Which of the following is true about the pathophysiology of this disease? It is**

    a. An autosomal dominant condition involving the reticuloendothelial system
    b. A gluten-induced enteropathy
    c. Increased mucus production of the endocrine glands
    d. An autosomal recessive disease involving the exocrine glands

3. **You evaluate that the mother of an infant with cystic fibrosis has understood your teaching about the pancreatic enzymes by which of the following statements?**

    a. "I give my baby enzymes between meals on an empty stomach."
    b. "I give my baby enzymes 30 minutes before she eats."
    c. "I give my baby enzymes with her food."
    d. "I give my baby enzymes 30 minutes after she eats."

4. **All of the following are risk factors for sudden infant death syndrome (SIDS) except**

    a. Sleeping in the prone position
    b. Sleeping in the supine position
    c. Having a sibling who died of SIDS
    d. History of prematurity

5. **The nurse recommends all of the following to prevent otitis media except**

   a. Feeding in an upright position
   b. Administration of the pneumococcal vaccine
   c. Hand washing
   d. Swabbing the ear canals regularly with a cotton swab

6. **RespiGam is most appropriate for which of the following patients?**

   a. Healthy young infant during a routine checkup
   b. Young infant with a history of bronchopulmonary dysplasia
   c. An infant during hospitalization with respiratory syncytial virus (RSV)
   d. The healthy 6-year-old sibling of a child with RSV

7. **A mother of a school-age child with moderate persistent asthma demonstrates understanding of medication administration by which of the following statements?**

   a. "I will administer the anti-inflammatory medication on a daily basis, whether it looks like he needs it or not."
   b. "I will administer cromolyn sodium (Intal) when he starts to have an asthma attack."
   c. "I will stop the oral corticosteroids as soon as his cold symptoms resolve."
   d. "I will administer the albuterol every night before he goes to sleep."

8. **You are reviewing diet teaching with a mother of a child with cystic fibrosis. Which of the following best describes the child's dietary requirements?**

   a. High fat, high calorie
   b. High protein, high calorie
   c. Low fat, low calorie
   d. Low protein, low calorie

9. Stridor is most commonly heard when assessing which of the following conditions?

    a. Croup
    b. Asthma
    c. Cystic fibrosis
    d. Pneumonia

10. A child, age 2, is brought to the emergency department after ingesting an unknown number of acetaminophen tablets about 30 minutes earlier. On entering the examination room, the child is crying and clinging to the mother. What data should the nurse obtain first?

    a. Heart rate, respiratory rate, and blood pressure
    b. Recent exposure to communicable diseases
    c. Number of immunizations received
    d. Height and weight

11. The greatest danger of acetaminophen overdose is which of the following?

    a. Metabolic acidosis
    b. Kidney failure
    c. Vomiting and diarrhea
    d. Liver failure

12. A preschool-age child underwent a tonsillectomy 4 hours ago. Which assessment finding would make the nurse suspect postoperative hemorrhage?

    a. Vomiting of dark brown emesis
    b. Refusal to drink clear fluids
    c. Decreased heart rate
    d. Frequent swallowing

13. A child, age 5, is diagnosed with mycoplasmal pneumonia and has a persistent productive cough. When assessing the child's respirations, the nurse should keep in mind that young children normally use which muscles to breathe?

    a. Accessory
    b. Thoracic
    c. Abdominal
    d. Intercostal

14. The parents of a school-age child with asthma express concern about letting the child participate in sports. What should the nurse tell the parents about the relationship between exercise and asthma?

    a. Asthma attacks are triggered by allergens, not exercise.
    b. The child should avoid exercise because it may trigger asthma attacks.
    c. Continuous activities, such as jogging, are less likely to trigger asthma than intermittent activities.
    d. Using prophylactic bronchodilators before the activity can prevent asthma attacks and enable the child to engage in most sports.

Answer Key

1.	b	8.	b
2.	d	9.	a
3.	c	10.	a
4.	b	11.	d
5.	d	12.	d
6.	b	13.	c
7.	a	14.	d

Chapter 11:
Renal and Genitourinary Conditions/Fluid and Electrolyte Balance

1. Which of the following best approximates the normal urine specific gravity for the infant?

    a. >1.030
    b. 1.021-1.030
    c. 1.010-1.020
    d. <1.010

2. Sara is a 10-month-old with dehydration. Her serum sodium is 137. You know that Sara has what type of dehydration?

    a. Isotonic
    b. Hypotonic
    c. Hypertonic
    d. Osmotic

3. Bobby is a 2-year-old admitted with hypertonic dehydration. Your priority nursing intervention for Bobby would be which of the following?

    a. Administer 0.9% normal saline via a peripheral IV at 1¼ maintenance fluid rate.
    b. Administer D5 ½ normal saline via a peripheral IV at 1¼ maintenance fluid rate.
    c. Perform daily weights.
    d. Perform neurologic assessments as needed.

4. Which of the following would be appropriate intervention for a child at risk for UTI?

    a. Have her drink carbonated beverages.
    b. Have her drink caffeinated beverages.
    c. Have her drink large amounts of clear fluids.
    d. Have her limit her intake of fluids to decrease stress on the kidneys.

5. **Which of the following would the nurse expect to see in the child with nephrotic syndrome?**

   a. Proteinuria and hypoalbuminemia
   b. Proteinuria and hyperalbuminemia
   c. Hypoglycosuria and hypoalbuminemia
   d. Hyperglycosuria and hyperalbuminemia

6. **Which of the following would the nurse expect to see in the 5-year-old male with nephrotic syndrome on a morning assessment?**

   a. Periorbital edema and abdominal ascites with anorexia
   b. Ankle edema and abdominal ascites with increased appetite
   c. Anemia and low urine specific gravity
   d. Urine that is clear with a low urine specific gravity

7. **You are the nurse performing discharge instructions with the parents of a child newly diagnosed with nephrotic syndrome. You evaluate that the mother understands proper dietary guidelines for her child by which of the following statements?**

   a. "I will give him foods that are high calorie, low protein, and high iron."
   b. "I will give him foods that are high calorie, high protein, and low salt."
   c. "I will give him foods that are low calorie, low protein, and low salt."
   d. "I will give him foods that are low calorie, high protein, and low potassium."

8. **You are the nurse caring for a newborn boy with undescended testicles. Which of the following would be the most appropriate information to share with his parents?**

   a. Typically, no intervention is done at this time; we will monitor the testes over the coming weeks to see if they descend on their own.
   b. Typically, surgery is at 12 weeks of life.
   c. Typically, prompt surgical correction of the problem is done to reduce complications related to sterility later on.
   d. The choice about whether or not to have surgical correction versus continuation of monitoring is up to the parents.

9. **Which of the following would the nurse expect to find in the history of an 8-month-old infant with hypospadias?**

    a. Circumcision
    b. Frequent urinary tract infection
    c. Pain on urination
    d. Kidney stones

10. **In a 3-month-old infant, fluid and electrolyte imbalance can occur quickly, primarily because an infant has**

    a. A lower percentage of body water than an adult
    b. A lower daily fluid requirement than an adult
    c. A more rapid heart rate than an adult
    d. Immature kidney function

11. **When caring for a 12-month-old infant with dehydration and metabolic acidosis, the nurse expects to see which of the following?**

    a. A reduced white blood cell count
    b. A decreased platelet count
    c. Apnea
    d. Tachypnea

12. **A 4-year-old girl has a urinary tract infection (UTI). When teaching the parents how to help her avoid recurrent UTIs, the nurse should emphasize which preventive measure?**

    a. Wiping her perineum from back to front after she uses the toilet
    b. Administering prophylactic antibiotics
    c. Giving her a warm bath for 15 minutes daily
    d. Making sure she avoids bubble baths

13. **In a pediatric patient, what is an early sign of acute renal failure?**

    a. Hypertension
    b. Decreased urine output
    c. Anemia
    d. Hematuria

Answer Key

1.	d	8.	a
2.	a	9.	b
3.	d	10.	d
4.	c	11.	d
5.	a	12.	d
6.	a	13.	d
7.	b		

Chapter 12:

Gastrointestinal Conditions

1. A newborn is suspected of having esophageal atresia and a tracheoesophageal fistula. What signs would the nurse notice?

    a. Excessive oral salivation
    b. No meconium passed
    c. Peristaltic waves
    d. Projectile vomiting

2. Celiac disease and cystic fibrosis are often confused. The diseases are similar because both

    a. Affect the lungs
    b. Affect the digestion of sugar
    c. Are eventually fatal
    d. Involve malabsorption

3. You are caring for a child in whom celiac disease has been newly diagnosed. Your parent-child education includes the avoidance of which of the following foods?

    a. Whole wheat bread
    b. Milk and milk products
    c. Beef and poultry
    d. Any sugar product

4. When assessing a child with intussusception the nurse is likely to note which of the following?

    a. Regurgitation
    b. Steatorrhea
    c. Projectile vomiting
    d. "Currant jelly" stools

5. Twenty-four hours after birth, a neonate has not passed meconium. The nurse suspects which condition?

    a. Celiac disease
    b. Intussusception
    c. Imperforate anus
    d. An abdominal wall defect

6. You are the nurse providing discharge instructions for parents of an infant in whom gastroesophageal reflux has been diagnosed. Which of the following would *not* be part of your teaching?

    a. Feeding the baby in an upright position
    b. Thickening feedings with rice cereal
    c. Placing the baby on his back to sleep
    d. Increasing the time between meals so that the empty stomach has time to rest

7. You are the nurse providing immediate postoperative care for a 2-month-old infant who has had a cleft lip repair. What intervention would the nurse plan to initiate?

    a. Place in flat prone position.
    b. Clean lip after feedings with alcohol.
    c. Keep child NPO for 24 hours post surgery.
    d. Keep the child propped in an infant seat/car seat.

8. A 4-week-old is suspected of having pyloric stenosis. Which of the following symptoms would you expect?

    a. Olive-size bulge in the abdomen
    b. Projectile vomiting of bile-tinged vomitus
    c. Malnutrition
    d. Inability to pass an NG tube

9. When caring for the child with inflammatory bowel disease, the nurse would expect all of the following except

    a. Projectile vomiting
    b. Bloody diarrhea
    c. Anemia
    d. Delayed growth

10. **When caring for the child in whom celiac disease has been recently diagnosed the nurse would expect all of the following except**

    a. Steatorrhea

    b. Failure to thrive

    c. Anemia

    d. Constipation

11. **When developing a postoperative plan of care for a toddler scheduled for cleft palate repair, the nurse should assign highest priority to which intervention?**

    a. Comforting the child as quickly as possible

    b. Maintaining the child in a supine position

    c. Restraining the child's arms at all times, using elbow restraints

    d. Assuring that the child is fed using a straw or nipple

12. **The physician suspects tracheoesophageal fistula in a 1-day-old neonate. Which nursing intervention is most appropriate for this child?**

    a. Avoid suctioning unless cyanotic.

    b. Give nothing by mouth.

    c. Elevate the neonate's head for 1 hour after feedings.

    d. Give the neonate only glucose water for the first 24 hours.

13. **A 9-month-old infant is admitted with diarrhea and dehydration. The nurse plans to assess the child's vital signs frequently. Which other action would provide the most important assessment information?**

    a. Measure the infant's head circumference.

    b. Obtain a stool specimen for analysis.

    c. Provide only clear fluids.

    d. Inspect the infant's anterior fontanel.

14. **You are the nurse is providing guidance for the parents of a 4-year-old with diarrhea. You recommend which of the following?**

    a. Caffeinated fluids
    b. Carbonated colas
    c. White rice
    d. Chocolate milk

15. **A toddler is brought to the emergency department with sudden onset of abdominal pain, vomiting, and stools that look like red currant jelly. To confirm intussusception, the suspected cause of these findings, the nurse expects the physician to order**

    a. A barium enema
    b. An MRI
    c. Nasogastric tube insertion
    d. Indwelling urinary (Foley) catheter insertion

16. **What is the most common assessment finding in a child with ulcerative colitis?**

    a. Intense abdominal cramps
    b. Profuse diarrhea
    c. Anal fissures
    d. Abdominal distention

Answer Key

1.	a	9.	a
2.	d	10.	d
3.	a	11.	c
4.	d	12.	b
5.	c	13.	d
6.	d	14.	c
7.	d	15.	a
8.	a	16.	b

Chapter 13:
Endocrine/Metabolic Conditions

1. The mother of a preschooler recently diagnosed with insulin-dependent diabetes mellitus makes an urgent call to the pediatrician's office. She says her child had an uncontrollable temper tantrum while playing and now is lethargic. The nurse should instruct the mother to take which action first?

   a. Obtain a urine sample and measure the glucose level.
   b. Force the child to drink orange juice.
   c. Measure the child's blood glucose level.
   d. This is typical of the age group and is not related to his diabetes.

2. When assessing a child with juvenile hypothyroidism, the nurse expects which finding?

   a. A high energy level
   b. Recent weight gain
   c. Diarrhea
   d. Tachycardia

3. A child with diabetes insipidus received desmopressin acetate. When evaluating for therapeutic effectiveness, the nurse would interpret which finding as a positive response to this drug?

   a. Decreased urine output
   b. Increased urine glucose level
   c. Decreased blood pressure
   d. Relief of nausea

4. Kia has type 1 diabetes mellitus and takes NPH and regular insulin in the morning. What must be included in the child's daily plan of care related to these medications?

   a. Check glucose level before going to sleep.
   b. Use lotion on the child's dry skin at the injection sites.
   c. Test the child's hemoglobin A1c.
   d. Assure that the child eats a snack with carbohydrates in the midafternoon.

5. **Hemoglobin A$_{1c}$ measures which of the following?**

    a. The current hemoglobin level
    b. The current glucose level
    c. The average blood glucose level over the past 3 months
    d. The extent to which complications will occur from the diabetes

6. **A normal blood glucose level is which of the following?**

    a. 80-120 mg/dl
    b. 60-80 mg/dl
    c. 120-140 mg/dl
    d. 40-60 mg/dl

7. **A rapid-acting insulin, such as Humalog or Lispro, should be given at what timeframe in relation to meals?**

    a. 30 minutes before eating
    b. Within a few minutes before eating
    c. 30 minutes after eating so you can assess what was eaten
    d. Between meals when the stomach is empty

8. **Which of the following is true about acanthosis nigricans?**

    a. It is a maculopapular rash caused by a reaction to taking too much insulin.
    b. It is a vascular complication of an inborn error of metabolism, such as PKU.
    c. It is the lipodystrophy that results from giving insulin in the same location.
    d. It is a thickening and hyperpigmentation of the skin of the neck due to type 2 diabetes.

Answer Key

1. b	5. c
2. b	6. a
3. a	7. b
4. d	8. d

Chapter 14:

Central Nervous System Conditions

1. **Cerebral palsy can be best defined as a**

    a. Congenital paralysis of voluntary muscles due to heredity
    b. Difficulty in controlling voluntary muscles due to brain damage
    c. Permanent loss of sensation due to cerebral pressure
    d. Muscle weakness and incoordination caused by mental retardation

2. **In cerebral palsy, intelligence**

    a. Is normal in more than half of those affected
    b. Is almost always subnormal
    c. Decreases with age
    d. Only goes to a certain level and stops

3. **In working with children who are blind, the nurse should**

    a. Repeat conversations
    b. Give the child extra attention
    c. Speak more frequently
    d. Speak before touching the child

4. **You are caring for 6-year-old Melissa, who is scheduled to start wearing a patch over her good eye because of amblyopia. How will you explain the reason for this practice to the parents?**

    a. It forces her to strengthen the muscles in the affected eye.
    b. They start by patching the strong eye, and then they will change and patch the weak eye.
    c. It allows the physician to see how the good eye responds to the stress.
    d. It is a way of seeing if the bad eye will get worse with strain.

5. **A child, age 3, with lead poisoning is admitted to the hospital for chelation therapy. The nurse must stay alert for which of the following adverse effects of lead poisoning or its treatment?**

    a. Anaphylaxis
    b. Fever and chills
    c. Seizures
    d. Congestive heart failure

6. **The nurse should begin screening for lead poisoning when a child reaches which age?**

    a. 6 months
    b. 12 months
    c. 4 years
    d. 8 years

7. **A newborn undergoes surgery to remove a myelomeningocele. To detect increased intracranial pressure (ICP) as early as possible, the nurse should stay alert for which postoperative finding?**

    a. Decreased urine output
    b. Increased heart rate
    c. Bulging fontanels
    d. Sunken eyeballs

8. **A neonate born 18 hours ago with meningomyelocele over the lumbosacral region is scheduled for corrective surgery. Preoperatively, what is the most important nursing goal?**

    a. Preventing infection
    b. Ensuring adequate hydration
    c. Providing adequate nutrition
    d. Preventing contracture deformity

9. **A child, age 5, with an intelligence quotient of 60 is admitted to the hospital for evaluation. When planning care, the nurse should keep in mind that this child is**

    a. Within normal range of intelligence
    b. Mildly retarded
    c. Moderately retarded
    d. Completely dependent on others for care

10. **A toddler is having a tonic-clonic major motor seizure. What should the nurse do first?**

    a.   Restrain the child.

    b.   Place a tongue blade in the child's mouth.

    c.   Remove objects from the child's surroundings.

    d.   Check the child's breathing.

11. **The parents of a 2-year-old child with chronic otitis media are concerned that the disorder has affected their child's hearing. Which behavior suggests that the child has a hearing impairment?**

    a.   Stuttering

    b.   Frequently pulling on his ears

    c.   Babbling rather than speaking

    d.   Playing alongside rather than interacting with peers

12. **When assessing a toddler, age 18 months, the nurse should interpret which of the following as a sign of a neurologic dysfunction?**

    a.   Positive gag reflex

    b.   Positive tonic neck reflex

    c.   Negative plantar grasp

    d.   Positive corneal reflex

Answer Key

1. b	5. c	9. b
2. a	6. b	10. d
3. d	7. c	11. c
4. a	8. a	12. b

Chapter 15:
Musculoskeletal Conditions

1. **When examining school-age and adolescent children, the nurse routinely screens for scoliosis. Which statement accurately summarizes how to perform this screening?**

    a. Have the child stand firmly on both feet and bend forward at the hips.
    b. Listen for a clicking sound as the child abducts the hips.
    c. Have the child run the heel of one foot down the shin of the other leg while standing.
    d. Have the child shrug the shoulders as the nurse applies pressure to the shoulders.

2. **Congenital hip dislocation is diagnosed in an infant. On assessment, the nurse expects to note**

    a. Symmetrical thigh gluteal folds
    b. Ortolani sign
    c. Increased hip abduction
    d. Femoral lengthening

3. **A child is admitted to the pediatric unit with a fracture of the hip. The physician orders Bryant's traction. The type of traction is**

    a. Skin traction applied to both legs, with the legs suspended 90° above the bed
    b. Skeletal traction applied to one leg
    c. Skin traction applied to an arm, suspending it above the bed
    d. Skeletal traction applied bilaterally to the lower extremities, at 45°

4. **A child with a fractured left femur receives a cast. A short time later, the nurse notices that the toes on the child's left foot are edematous. Which nursing action would be most important?**

    a. Applying ice to the foot
    b. Massaging the toes
    c. Elevating the foot of the bed
    d. Placing the child on the right side

5. **Which type of fracture in a young child would have the greatest impact on the child's future growth?**

    a. A greenstick fracture
    b. Fracture of the fibula
    c. Fracture to the tibia
    d. Fracture to the epiphyseal plate

6. **What assessments would you make of a 3-year-old with a diagnosis of Duchenne's muscular dystrophy?**

    a. Lethargy, pallor, and a low hemoglobin
    b. Uses his hands to push himself off the floor from a sitting position
    c. Mild mental retardation or cognitive delay
    d. Seizure activity

Answer Key

1. a
2. b
3. a
4. c
5. d
6. b

Chapter 16:
Dermatologic Conditions

1. **To treat atopic dermatitis, the physician prescribes a topical application of hydrocortisone cream twice daily. After medication instruction by the nurse, which statement by the parent indicates effective teaching?**

    a. "I will spread a thick coat of hydrocortisone cream on the affected area and will wash the area once daily."
    b. "I will gently scrape the skin before applying the cream to promote absorption."
    c. "I will avoid using soap and water on the affected area and will apply the cream on this area frequently."
    d. "I will wash the affected area twice daily before applying a thin layer of the cream."

2. **Which nursing diagnosis takes highest priority for a child in the early stages of burn recovery?**

    a. Risk for infection
    b. Impaired physical mobility
    c. Body image disturbance
    d. Constipation

3. **For a child with a circumferential chest burn, what is the most important factor for the nurse to assess?**

    a. Wound characteristics
    b. Body temperature
    c. Breathing pattern
    d. Heart rate

4. **Baby Daniel has diaper rash. Your recommendation to the mother is which of the following?**

    a. Change to using cloth diapers with rubber pants rather than disposable diapers.
    b. Remove the diaper for periods of time to expose to the air.
    c. Wash vigorously with half-strength hydrogen peroxide, at least every 2 hours.
    d. Change the type of formula to a soy-based formula.

5. **Which of the following is true about a pediculosis infestation in school-age children?**

   a. They indicate a lack of hygiene on the part of the child or family.
   b. Nits are live lice and can jump from head to head.
   c. Lice attach to the hair shafts close to the scalp so the lice can feed on the scalp.
   d. Lice cause no symptoms, so the nurse must screen all school-age children.

6. **Which of the following is true about poison ivy?**

   a. The lesions that result are contagious to others.
   b. Eruptions can be prevented by showering with soap immediately after contact.
   c. The lesions can cause serious neurologic consequences if not treated.
   d. Animals cannot transfer the oils from their contact with poison ivy to humans.

Answer Key

1.	d	4.	b
2.	a	5.	c
3.	c	6.	b

Chapter 17:
Psychiatric and Psychological Conditions

1. **What statement by a child's parent would be revealing about an abusing parent's personality?**

    a. My kid cries all of the time.
    b. My kid never smiles at me; he doesn't like me.
    c. She's such a fussy eater.
    d. I can't wait until this kid sleeps through the night.

2. **A 9-month-old infant is brought to the emergency department for bronchiolitis. Which of the following supports a diagnosis of child abuse?**

    a. The child is crying.
    b. The child is sitting quietly in the mother's lap.
    c. The mother refuses to stay with the child during her blood work.
    d. Chest X-ray shows multiple healed fractured ribs.

3. **A child, age 4, is hospitalized because of alleged sexual abuse. What is the best nursing intervention for this child?**

    a. Avoid touching the child.
    b. Prevent the suspected abuser from visiting the child.
    c. Provide play situations that allow disclosure.
    d. Discourage the child from talking about what happened.

4. **A toddler is hospitalized with multiple injuries. Although the parent states that the child fell down the stairs, the child's history and physical findings suggest abuse as the cause of the injuries. What should the nurse do first?**

    a. Refer the parent to a support group, such as Parents Anonymous.
    b. Report the incident to the proper authorities.
    c. Prepare the child for foster care placement.
    d. Restrict the parent from the child's room.

5. An adolescent is admitted with a tentative diagnosis of clinical depression. Which assessment finding is most significant in confirming the diagnosis?

    a. Irritability
    b. Sadness
    c. Weight gain
    d. Low exercise tolerance

6. A girl, age 15, is brought to the pediatrician's office by her mother, who is concerned about her daughter's dramatic weight loss over the past 6 months and she is now below the 3rd percentile of weight for height. The nurse suspects that the child has anorexia nervosa. Besides weight loss, nursing assessment of this patient is likely to reveal

    a. Insomnia
    b. Dysphagia
    c. Diarrhea
    d. Amenorrhea

7. A girl, age 13, with anorexia nervosa is admitted to the hospital for IV fluid therapy and nutritional management. She says she is worried that the IV fluids will make her gain weight. Which nursing diagnosis is most appropriate?

    a. Noncompliance
    b. Body image disturbance
    c. Dysfunctional grieving
    d. Anticipatory grieving

8. A teenager is admitted for treatment of bulimia nervosa. When developing the plan of care, the nurse anticipates including interventions that address which metabolic disorders?

    a. Hypoglycemia
    b. Hyponatremia
    c. Metabolic alkalosis
    d. Metabolic acidosis

9. **Mark has ADHD and has been prescribed stimulants. His father is opposed to stimulant use and states that the physician is just "drugging" his child. Your best response is**

    a.   "You will need to speak to the physician about your concern."

    b.   "It does seem odd that your child would be ordered a stimulant when he is already hyperactive. I will check on that."

    c.   "The stimulant will actually treat his other comorbid psychiatric conditions."

    d.   "The stimulants help most children with ADHD to focus better."

10. **Rebecca, age 14, has an auditory processing learning disability. You need her to give you a clean-catch urine sample. What is your best way to have her understand the directions?**

    a.   Demonstrate what you want her to do with a model.

    b.   Give her the directions verbally, but very slowly, so she can process them.

    c.   Know that you will have to catheterize her to get a clean sample.

    d.   Go into the bathroom with her and clean her perineum and hold the cup.

11. **What are classic features you would expect to see in a child with autism?**

    a.   Eating of nonfood substances and having an imaginary companion

    b.   Impaired social interactions and fascination with spinning objects

    c.   Bipolar behaviors and speech impediments

    d.   Small for age and learning disabilities in reading and mathematics

Answer Key

1. b	5. b	9. d
2. d	6. d	10. a
3. c	7. b	11. b
4. b	8. c	

Chapter 18:
Issues and the Law

1. **The Individuals with Disabilities Education Improvement Act (IDEA) guarantees what rights to children with disabilities?**

    a. If otherwise qualified, they must be accepted or hired into a program or job
    b. Privacy regarding medical information
    c. Free and appropriate public education in the least restrictive environment
    d. Civil rights related to access to transportation and public buildings

Answer Key

1. c

Index

T

U

V

W